Fernanda Cabral Schveitzer

Mariana Cabral Schveitzer

SELF-CARE

A dynamic approach to integral health

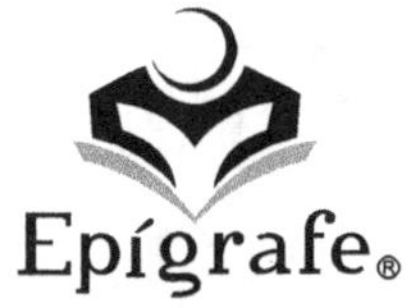

Epígrafe®

Foz do Iguaçu – Paraná – Brazil

2022

Editorial production: Ernani Brito.

Illustrations (cover and core): Jéssica Zanovelo Fogaça.

Translation: Fernanda Lise and Flávia Lise Garcia.

Revision: Jaclyn Cowen, Victoria Chbane and Daniel Hiram Zengotita.

International Catalog Data in publication (CIP)

S397S	Schveitzer, Fernanda Cabral
	Self-care: a dynamic approach to integral health. / Fernanda Cabral Schveitzer and Mariana Cabral Schveitzer; [preface Maria Júlia Paes da Silva]. - Foz do Iguaçu: Epígrafe, 2022.
	282 p.
	Includes bibliography. ISBN 978-65-87816-19-7
	1. Consciential health. 2. Conscientiology. I. Silva, Maria Júlia Paes da. II. Title.
	CDU 133

Tatiana Lopes CRB 9/1524

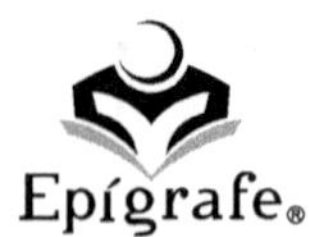

EPIGRAFE EDITORIAL AND GRAPHIC LTD.
Cosmoética Street, 1635 – Cognópolis
CEP: 85856-852 – Foz do Iguaçu-PR
Phone: 55 (45) 98419-0824
Virtual store: www.shopcons.com.br
www.epigrafe.com.br

SELF-CARE

A dynamic approach
to integral health

Dedication

To those consciousnesses committed
to care and self-care.

Acknowledgments

To our parents, Fátima and Tarcísio, we express our gratitude for the practical lessons of care and for the adventures of life we shared with you. We discovered the world together and learned a great deal in living with the Cabral-Schveitzer Family. *We love you very much.*

On this journey we expanded our family: Fernanda and Cesar, Mariana and Victor Hugo. We thank you for the support and love that has guided our journey together. Thanks also to the family that grew up with you, who are now our fathers- and mothers-in-law, brothers- and sisters-in-law, cousins, nephews and nieces, which multiplied the affection.

To Laura, our youngest sister, our gratitude for showing us the importance of love and forgiveness.

We would also like to thank Dr. Waldo Vieira (*in memoriam*), for the conscientiological teachings, the extraphysical helpers for the opportunities of interassistance and the AIEC, ECTOLAB, IIPC, Intercons, Interparadigmas and UNICIN teams for the opportunities of growth through volunteering.

To the dedicated professionals of the Epigrafe Publishing House Gisele Salles, Rosemary Salles and Ernani Brito and portuguese edition reviewers Giséle Razera and Cesar Cordioli, our gratitude for their efforts in reviewing and publishing this work.

Thank you to Professor Maria Julia! Her loving and encouraging words filled the Portuguese language preface and our hearts.

Our gratitude to caregivers, to the therapists and health professionals who, through their personal example, assisted and taught us different ways of caring.

Mariana would also like to thank the following people: the Knecht Family who welcomed me to Iowa City, USA, with open arms, Professor Margarete Sandelowski for her research guidance at Chapel Hill, USA, and the dear graduate advisors: Professors Vânia Backes, Elma Zoboli and Marta Melleiro. To Marcelo Fabian Oliva who guided me down the path of traditional Chinese medicine in Brazil, China and Cuba. To the health professionals who opened the doors for my work with complementary therapies, especially, Maria Tereza Andreola and Desireé Souza. To my colleagues from the CUIDAR [CARE] Research Group, and from the Preventive Medicine Department at the Paulista Medical School of Unifesp, for their reception and the experience of doing projects together. *Together we go further.*

Fernanda would like to express gratitude to her colleagues and professors throughout this health journey: I would especially like to thank Professor Mário Steindel, for introducing me to this path of research. To Itaipu's health team, from before and now, for their dedication and for showing me that the practice of care has many styles and ways. *Experience is the best teacher.*

The authors would also like to thank translators Fernanda Lise and Flávia Lise Garcia, reviewers Victoria Chbane, Daniel Zengotita and Jaclyn Cowen, for their meticulous work of translating this book into the English language, enabling us to expand the scope of the developed research.

Finally, we especially thank our patients, because, in the search to better care for them, we developed the knowledge we present in this book.

Gratitude: Reversed generosity.
Waldo Vieira (1932–2015)[1:509].

Contents

PART I

Development of Health Knowledge

PART II

Development of Care Practices

Preface to the English Language Edition

Welcome to the self-care journey. Self-care is the experienced interaction of self-knowledge, understanding of health models, and the good use of available therapeutic resources and practices. It is a practice of self-connection and of reinventing yourself by expanding your understanding of the world and yourself, your interests and purpose in life.

The **objective** of translating this work into English is to meet three demands: the first, to present the construction of the self-care triad and the FEMA method to an international audience; the second, to promote health care practices that are carried out in Brazil, especially in the Unified Health System (Sistema Único de Saúde – SUS); and the third, to publicize the consciential paradigm and consciential health.

The **authors** of this book are sisters who grew up in southern Brazil, immersed in a syncretic culture, with a predominance of modern Western health, yet surrounded by a variety of experiences of other health models, whether in the care provided to them and their families, in the early stages of life; during the health training they chose to follow; or even in the health practices they chose to use in search of personal harmony.

Dr. Fernanda Schveitzer is a physician (Federal University of Santa Catarina – UFSC), who specializes in occupational medicine (Brazilian Medical Association/National Association of Occupational Medicine – AMB/ANAMT) and works in occupational health management. At the moment, she is the occupational medicine manager at Itaipu Binacional. Along with her medical studies, she has dedicated herself to experimenting with and offering alternative health approaches and therapeutic practices, for her own self-care and that of her family, friends and patients. She is also a volunteer and researcher of conscientiology, focusing on the subject areas of consciential health and the evolution of consciousness.

Dr. Mariana Schveitzer is a nurse (UFSC), holds a Post-Doctorate (School of Nursing at the University of São Paulo – EEUSP), PhD in Science (EEUSP-Catholic University of Portugal – UCP), Master of Nursing (UFSC), is specialized in Public Health (UFSC) and Acupuncture (Faculty of Health Technology – CIEPH-Shandong University), and has completed significant additional training in complementary therapies. She worked as an acupuncture and holistic therapist, and currently holds the role of Assistant Professor at the Preventive Medicine Department at the Paulista Medical School at the Federal University of São Paulo (UNIFESP), in addition to conducting research related to human aspects of care, scientific methodology and complementary therapies. She is a volunteer and researcher of conscientiology, with an emphasis on the subject areas of embracement and instruments of conscientiological research.

Together, the authors have built an **integrative health care** approach, supported by the multiple health models and therapeutic offers available, capable of adapting to the context and perspectives of the world experienced by each person, while supported by the self-care triad.

The **self-care triad** consists of 1) the knowledge of oneself and one's health reference (self-knowledge), 2) an understanding of the production of knowledge and health technologies (cosmovision), and 3) the good use of techniques and practices in health (resources). These three factors are related to and mutually influence the production of personal well-being and can be applied in practice through the use of the FEMA method, with the tools being available in the book and at www.autocuidado.org for free download.

The **FEMA method** was developed by the authors, based on more than ten years of research and clinical practice. Its four stages were initially conceived in the English language from the words: 1) *Find*: needs or discomfort; 2) *Embrace*: feelings and thoughts; 3) *Move*: to a new benchmark of well-being and 4) *Again*: restart the self-care cycle whenever necessary.

The authors' proposal is not to define the best **path**, but in fact to modify the logic of the construction of care, with an appreciation of technologies of different rationales and understandings in health, in constant interaction, to learn how to take care of oneself and others, in an integrative way.

The concept of self-care presented in this book is the result of a unique **context** of experiences that coexist in Brazilian culture, which provide a dialogue of different types of knowledge and paradigms of health. Understanding this work and its contribution to personal and collective health and well-being involves understanding the context in which it was produced:

A. The blending of ethnic groups, races, creeds and health understandings of a population distributed throughout its continental territory. Its strong popular wisdom in using traditional therapies, passed down by tradition in families and social circles, until the present time, derived from indigenous native cultures and immigrants, which include the use of herbs, teas, compresses, bottles, massages, blessings, among others.

B. A health system that proposes to provide universal and free access to the whole population and which coexists with the provision of private health, whose access is restricted only to those who can afford it, demonstrating the great challenge that is present in the promotion of health and disease prevention nowadays.

The Brazilian Unified Health System (SUS) spans across the entire national territory, serving a public of more than 150 million people (base year 2019), and since 2006, SUS has been incorporating humanizing practices and Integrative and Complementary Practices in Health (Práticas Integrativas e Complementares em Saúde – PICS).

Humanizing practices recover the respect and ethics in the relationships between professionals and patients, thereby increasing the quality and satisfaction of care. They include bonding, extended listening, embracing, integrality and protagonism. These practices can be related to the Patient-Centered Care proposal, in the sense that they value different types of knowledge and recover the individuality of the human being and their autonomy in the care process.

PICS include rationales, health practices and complementary therapies of Traditional, Complementary and Integrative Medicines (TCIM), such as: traditional Chinese medicine, acupuncture, ayurveda medicine, yoga, and meditation. The World Health Organization (WHO) uses the term TCIM and, in Brazil, we use the term PICS to talk about the inclusion of these practices in SUS. In this book we will use the term complementary therapies as a correspondent of PICS. Currently, there are 29 practices included in the National Policy of Integrative and Complementary Practices in Health. In SUS, complementary therapies are mostly offered in Primary Health Care, the patient's gateway to the Health Care Services Network. In the private market, the number of complementary therapies offered in the national territory is even greater and continues to grow.

Since 2018, the Virtual Health Library on Traditional, Complementary and Integrative medicines (VHL TCIM) has been presenting research results and demonstrating the effects of these practices through interactive maps. This project is the result of a partnership between the Brazilian Ministry of Health, the Brazilian Academic Consortium of Integrative Health and the Latin American and Caribbean Center on Health Sciences Information, also known by its original name, Regional Library of Medicine (Biblioteca Regional de Medicina – BIREME), of the Pan American Health Organization/World Health Organization (PAHO/WHO). The TCIM Evidence Maps project was born from the need to identify evidence among the more than 1 million scientific studies available in the VHL TCIM and other databases.

C. The emergence in Brazil of the science of conscientiology, proposed by the Brazilian physician and researcher Waldo Vieira (1932–2015), which is dedicated to the investigation of the integral consciousness. Among the assumptions of this neoscience are the holosoma (different bodies with which the consciousness manifests itself), multidimensionality (multiple dimensions of manifestation), multiexistentiality (the set of successive human existences) and the thosene (the indissociable expression of thought, sentiment and energy). The approach to health from a conscientiological perspective, its principles and practical applications in everyday life, also make up the content of this work.

The confluence of this knowledge and experiences motivated the authors to recover the meaning of **care**, in order to help understand what should be considered to achieve self-care and integral health, whether for ourselves, for the people around us, or for those we assist professionally.

It should be noted that this book does not aim to replace the services and treatments provided by health professionals, therapists and caregivers. The information contained here is intended to complement the **assistance** and broaden one's view on the construction of self-care.

Throughout the chapters you will find notes to contextualize definitions and practices in health, in addition to the **glossary** that will help the reader to understand the conscientiological neo-concepts presented in the book.

We wish you a pleasant reading!
The authors.

Preface to the Portuguese Language Edition

"What was the dog's name?"

Have you ever imagined an anamnesis (medical history) starting with this question? Indeed, what does it have to do with a medical history? If you, dear reader, started to smile when reading this sentence, maybe you have understood and share the author's opinion that the provision of care is much more than what has been practiced in many institutions, by many professionals, and by many people! Throughout the book we will provide a context to this question: *"what was the dog's name?"*

This book you have in your hands will help you to reflect on the best way to take care of your health: yours, mine, ours. To this end, the book exposes the myths of current science, questions its neutrality and independence, and provides tips for identifying opportunities to expand your self-knowledge, self-awareness and self-scientificity. This is no small task, but Fernanda and Mariana have the ability to present their ideas in a clear, didactic manner, with the use of poetry, philosophy, suggested films, books and... many questions.

We know that the brain likes questions, so reading this book flows. They refer to Michel Foucault in Chapter 5: *"There are times in life when the question of knowing if one can think differently than one thinks, and perceive differently than one sees, is absolutely necessary if one is to go on looking and reflecting at all."*

I confess that the invitation to write this Preface, in addition to being a great honor, surprised me; but, being a nurse, I spent much of my life reflecting, learning, experiencing the meaning of care, which models and practices to adopt in the face of so many options, to serve as an instrument in the therapeutic process and to qualify my own life, in its multiple dimensions and roles. It is to have attention, intention, and awareness regarding the physical, emotional, mental, energetic, and spiritual aspects. To integrate what can be integrated; whether it has a western or eastern origin. To combine ancient healing systems with modern Western medicine.

There is a central aspect of the book that makes us, the readers, feel very valued: the importance of our own experiences! Self-research to achieve self-healing. The authors used the reference of consciential health! We know that the consciousness is a current scientific challenge and conscientiological research urges readers/researchers to develop critical thinking about what is subjective and indissociable, by proposing a way of doing science by yourself and about yourself, for the benefit of all and the Universe itself. Do you want a more thought-provoking question than that?

Reflecting on our experiences as patients of health services, we understand the importance of keeping our permanent attention on models and practices that impact quality, which broadens the gaze to the human being that.... the person is much more than their disease! Labeling someone with a disease is to reduce them, to deny all of their (our) potential for creativity and life.

During our time of "experientially" living a pandemic and while reading this book, I remembered a current educator that I love very much: Edgar Morin. According to him, *by sacrificing the essential for the urgent, one ends up forgetting the urgency of the essential*. The essential requires discipline, commitment, involvement and will. Reading this book can help us remember the essentials, for life goes on.

Thank you, Fernanda! Thank you, Mariana! For broadening our gaze, for stimulating us to analyze how much we take ownership of our own self-care and, therefore, our own life. Always take care with love; it is the way.

By the way, the name of my puppy was Fluffy. She lived for 17 physical years in our family. Today she lives in my heart, in a place called gratitude.

> *"...the truth is not in the setting out nor in the arriving: it comes to us in the middle of the journey."*
> (The Devil to Pay in the Backlands. J. Guimarães Rosa)

Pleasant reading, dear readers!
Have fun with questions and life.

Maria Júlia Paes da Silva

Retired full Prof. of University of São Paulo School of Nursing - EEUSP; Vipassana Meditator; practitioner of *Tai Chi Chuan;* author of the book: O amor é o caminho: maneiras de cuidar [Love is the way: Ways to care], Ed. Loyola, among others.

Introduction

Health care is a practice as old as humanity. It already existed long before dictionaries defined its meaning, science conceived its paradigms, universities taught their craft, services standardized clinical protocols, or laboratories researched diagnoses and cures. The evolution of health care has accompanied history, transforming itself together with societies.

Different paradigms and worldviews interfere in health practices and research that are carried out to categorize, identify and treat the most diverse diseases. Much more than theoretical discussions, different health visions integrate the bases of what professionals are able to offer and what patients learn to expect. However, the encounter of these different types of knowledge does not guarantee meeting the person's needs in an integral context, nor the satisfaction of the professionals involved in the care.

Recovering the meaning of care is the purpose of this book, in order to help in understanding what needs to be considered to achieve self-care and integral health, whether for ourselves, for the people around us, or for those we assist professionally. It is a work dedicated to patients, family members, professionals, therapists, caregivers, and everyone interested in better understanding and improving their health and care practice.

This book is an invitation to reflect on the following questions, among others distributed throughout the chapters:

1. *What is the best way to take care of my health?*

2. *Which models and practices of health care should I adopt, among many others available?*

3. *What challenges and opportunities does my health condition bring me?*

4. *How can I research myself and develop a strategy to optimize my own self-care and the people I assist?*

5. *How can I obtain more self-knowledge and self-awareness through self-research? And how can I support other people in this construction?*

To achieve these goals, we recover the development of health knowledge and health care practices, present integrative and complementary therapies (traditional Chinese medicine, yoga, meditation, among others), humanizing practices (embracing, listening, amplified clinic, among others), consciential health and self-research, to diversify and qualify the assistance.

The proposal is not to define the best path, but, in fact, to modify the logic behind the construction of health care, with an appreciation of technologies from different rationales and understandings of health, to learn how to take care of yourself and others, in an integrative manner. In this process, it is important to recover the objectives of care, the roles played by patients and professionals, and to expand the tools used to improve health care and stimulate autonomy, self-knowledge, and self-awareness.

However, it should be noted that this book does not aim to replace the services and treatments provided by health professionals, therapists and caregivers, but rather to complement the assistance and broaden your understanding of self-care.

To amplify your reading experience, we suggest you adopt five postures:

1. Pay attention to the initial and final questions of each chapter, looking to answer them as the concepts are presented. Reflections are an integral part of the process.

2. Direct your reading from the summary words or expressions of each paragraph, highlighted in bold to help fix your attention and facilitate understanding.

3. Deepen your knowledge of the topics through the indicated references of videos, books and articles, which can broaden your insights.

4. Consider the cases presented, which are real, although the identities are safeguarded by fictitious names.

5. Consult the glossary for any questions concerning the neologisms presented in this book.

This work is organized into two parts: The first is dedicated to the development of knowledge about health, divided into five chapters; and the second addresses the development of care practices, divided into four chapters.

The first part presents a historical review of health and care concepts, the main paradigms, integrative health and consciential health, besides the development of science and research about health and the consciousness, in order to provoke a critical posture regarding scientific discoveries.

In the first chapter, we address the development of health conceptions and the movements that established the predominant health models in Western health. In the second, we differentiate between traditional, complementary and alternative health practices, highlighting the continued expansion of these movements in search of new forms of health and care. In the third chapter, we characterize health from the consciential paradigm, introducing the neoscience conscientiology, which studies the consciousness from an integral perspective, and we list the principles of consciential health.

Chapter Four shows how health knowledge is produced through different paradigms, and how the research developed modifies the care and assistance provided. It explains the challenge that science faces in innovating itself, due to the way it is structured, and it reinforces the importance of including subjectivity in health research. It elucidates the renovating potential of qualitative and mixed research designs, and research into alternative and complementary practices, by enabling the integration of subjectivity into care.

Chapter Five presents the indissociable connections between health and the consciousness that are expressed through their personal traits, temperament and essence. It emphasizes the impact of these relationships on the provision of health and on the construction of care, and the complexity of researching the consciousness, in the sciences in general and from the perspective of conscientiology.

The second part examines the care offered by health professionals and services and the expectations of patients and society. It invites the reader to recognize and reflect on their actions and practices of health and care through the FEMA method, developed from the experience of these authors, which promotes self-research.

Chapter Six discusses how the models to control and eliminate diseases have become limited, especially when they distance the patient from the care process. Moreover, it proposes integrative health care with the use of light technologies, such as embracing, listening, empathy and interprofessional collaboration, as well as the means and actions to promote consciential health.

In chapter Seven, we present the challenge of health practices to incorporate autonomy and integrality. We highlight the role of the patients in the therapeutic project, to recover their motivation for self-care, using the amplified clinic, the anti-protocol, the singular therapeutic project and multidimensional care. And we exemplify the complexity of incorporating these values through the case of pain.

In chapter Eight, we elucidate the factors that influence the development of self-conviviality and the elements that make up the self-care triad. By combining health knowledge with our personal and professional experience, we create the FEMA method as a tool to facilitate the promotion of self-care in the search for integral health. The FEMA method, or the dynamic and continuous self-care cycle, is organized in four stages: *Find-Embrace-Move-Again*. Each step is described in detail in this chapter and we offer tools that favor its application by the person or with professional support, as well as demonstrate a real case of using the method.

The last chapter invites the reader to reflect and research themselves. It proposes self-research as a tool to broaden your self-knowledge and self-awareness, so as to qualify your self-care, and experience daily life with more lucidity and applied scientificity.

The book demonstrates the process of growth and self-care experienced by the authors, from the conception of new ideas related to new paradigms to their practical application with yourself and others. Through this dynamic approach, self-experimentation and self-research provide personal recycling and the ability to reach new ways of living, which in turn, constitutes the ascending cyclical process of self-evolution.

We seek to develop an inter-paradigmatic approach between Western, integrative and consciential health in this book, however, without the desire of exhausting the subject. The purpose is to reflect on the role of professionals and each person in the promotion of health, care and self-research, based on different paradigms, in constant interaction. The authors await the weighted contributions from other researchers in the continuous exercise of integral health. We wish you all good reading!

> *"the publication of a work always brings the award of invaluable and free heterocriticism."*
> Waldo Vieira (1932–2015)[1:422][Translation].

PART I

Development of Health Knowledge

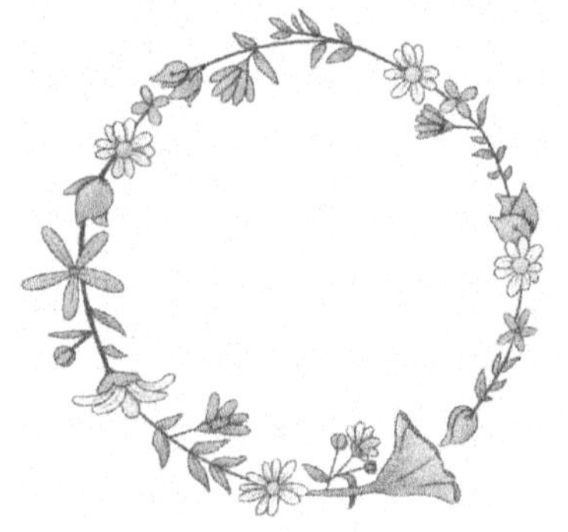

Chapter 1
Conceptions of Health and Care

"Everything, for us, is in our concept of the world. To modify our concept of the world is to modify the world for us, or simply to modify the world, since it will never be, for us, anything but what it is for us." [Translation]

Fernando Pessoa (1888–1935)

When you think about **health**, what first comes to mind? And when you think about **care**? The purpose of this chapter is to broaden one's *understanding of these concepts* through a *brief historical review.*

Our language is modulated by the concepts and conceptions that we absorb from the world, and what we use to communicate, interact and build knowledge. To recover the **meaning** of health and care that we adopt today requires reflecting on how each person thinks about such concepts, until they begin to compose their own personal conceptions.

For starters, what is a **concept**? A concept is a term, used to describe concrete or abstract phenomena, experiences or realities, through words. The construction of a concept is based on the pre-vailing philosophical, theoretical and political conceptions at a given time, and it is therefore not possible to approach a concept without reflecting on its history[2].

A **conception** is what we conceive in our mind from concepts, ideas and opinions[3]. It's a way to see or feel something. Health conceptions reflect the social, economic, political and cultural situation of different people and are therefore dependent on the time period, place, social class, individual values, and scientific, religious and philosophical currents[4]. With this, we can understand that there is a wide variety of conceptions about health and care, which interfere both in the way care is practiced and in public health policies. This variety justifies the fact that some concepts are valid for certain periods and then criticized and even replaced.

The provision of **care** is one of the oldest practices in history. For thousands of years, the practice of care did not depend on a health system, much less belong to a profession. It concerned anyone who helped others to continue their lives in relation to the group, being guided by two situations: ensuring life and holding back death[5].

However, care practices have evolved over time from **changes** in multiple contexts. In the social sphere, for example, an attempt was made to define who should have the role of caregiver: whether it should be men, women, young people, the elderly, of what social class and with what background and profession. In economics, it means to quantify how much it costs: how to value the spent time, dedication and structure. In the cultural context, to define how care is recognized: what financial and social values are attributed to it. In technology, what is the best way to do it: with what methods, techniques and equipment. And as such, care was divided and spread out into different tasks and professions.

The way a person receiving care is seen has also undergone profound changes. If it once focused on the integrality of the individual, the person was gradually isolated, parceled, split and separated from the social and collective dimensions that composed them, especially in the West. The practice of care, over time, became treating the **disease**[5]. In this process, general care to maintain life, such as eating, sleeping, exercising and relating to others, that was developed from popular wisdom, was gradually replaced by scientifically proven knowledge in many cultures.

The historical transformation that has occurred by the act of care can be perceived, for example, at different **moments** in the development of the medical profession in the West, as organized by Professor Nelson Filice de Barros[6]:

1. **Empirical medicine:** notions of care and prevention are acquired from routine observations, with an individual resolution of health problems.

2. **Magical-religious medicine:** there is recognition of the individual caregiver and the role of the healer, who explains the illness process and promotes healing.

3. **Hippocratic medicine:** medical care incorporates the theoretical matrix of hippocratic medicine, encompassing semiology, prognosis and therapy.

4. **Medicine in the Middle Ages:** the patient is recognized as a person in the purification process, carried out through pain, suffering and illness.

5. **Medicine in modernity:** establishes the division between scientific knowledge and common sense; health is compartmentalized into specialties, systems and organs, that increasingly rely on the use of measuring instruments.

Patients and health professionals can adopt different conceptions of health and care influenced by these moments. A patient who perceives their illness as a punishment approaches care from the Medieval perspective and still presents this perspective today. When attending to this patient, a professional can take the opportunity to broaden the patient's understanding and the way in which they relate to their health, or they can choose to disregard this information. When addressing the patient's conception of health, they may even disqualify the patient, incorporate it into an *as it is* therapeutic proposal, or interact with it so that the patient can revisit it and gain new meaning from it. Thus, on a daily basis, professionals act as **multipliers** of health knowledge and models, both for patients and their colleagues.

Such conceptions and models integrate an even greater set of established assumptions, theories, methods and procedures that characterize a science. Known as a **paradigm,** this concept expresses the matrix or model that structures and governs a specific scientific field at a given place and time in history. In practice, paradigms define the *lenses* we use to observe the reality around us, conduct research, value knowledge and endorse what is *recognized as scientific*.

Emerging from modernity, the health sciences developed fundamental characteristics, such as unicausality, mechanism and objectivity which stimulated what became known as the paradigm of **modern medicine**[a], also called a biomedical model.

---

a The term modern medicine adopted in this book refers to modern Western medicine, also called allopathic medicine, biomedicine, conventional medicine or mainstream medicine. Some authors also call it contemporary Western medicine. The expression composed with the biomedical term used in this work (such as biomedical model, biomedical knowledge or biomedical practice) also refers to this conception, which does not refer to the area of Biomedicine training.

The discovery of several disease-causing microorganisms and the development of bacteriology and antibiotics have helped to consolidate the notion of the **unicausality** of diseases in the dominant medical practice[6].

By interpreting diseases and cures as mechanical occurrences, that result from a physical-chemical interaction, medicine absorbs the **mechanicism** from physics and biology. This reduction excludes the interference of the patient's subjectivity, their history and context of life, from the general understanding of what health is. For the social scientist Marcos Queiroz[7], this was how medicine emerged as a modern science. The therapeutic act is explained by the chemical or physical intervention in different parts and structures of the organism, with the aim of eliminating the disease. The concentration of the scientific gaze to increasingly smaller parts of the biological body, eventually led to the loss of the patient being approached as an integrated human being.

Thus, there is a **separation** between the disease's objectiveness and the patient's subjectiveness and also a **split** between medical theory and practice, because, while the former becomes precise and objective, the latter remains uncertain and fallible[8]. Such reductionism in modern medicine resulted in limitations to the biomedical model[6], in which three aspects regarding its practical application stand out:

1. A low ability to **share** its knowledge with the population and to act in conjunction with other forms of care.

2. An unequal relationship with the physician presenting a style of **domination** in relation to the patient, justified by the autonomy and technical competence of the professional.

3. The **passive** and subordinate participation of the patient, by excluding his knowledge, representation, uses and popular customs in relation to the health-disease process.

The appreciation of objectivity in biomedical science, as opposed to the subjectivity of being, led to a **crisis** in modern medicine, not just in relation to knowledge itself, but in relation to the ethical, political, pedagogical and social dimensions inherent in the health care context[8,9].

Concomitant to this process, the provision of **care** also transforms with social changes and the emergence of science. The history and evolution of care can be organized in three different moments in the West as proposed by the French historian and nurse Marie-Françoise Collière[5]:

1. Practices of women who provide **care**, from the earliest times in human history to the Middle Ages.

2. Care practices of women recognized as **caregivers**, from prostitutes to nuns, from the Middle Ages to the end of the 19th century.

3. Female **nursing**, as a profession with a defined moral and technical role, from the beginning of the 20th century to the end of the 60's.

The practice of care has **differentiated** between women and men throughout human history[5]. Women were predominantly involved in care practices to ensure the maintenance of life, especially those concerning childbirth and the sick person. Men repaired the injured body, which often required physical strength to dominate people in a state of agitation, delirium or madness.

This distinction explains how women became nurses and men became physicians, surgeons and nurses in prisons, leper colonies and asylums. The division of labor between **genders** was not so much a result of scientific advances, but of the very structuring of society, which attributes some forms of care and types of knowledge to one gender, to the detriment of the other[5].

During the Middle Ages, the woman caregiver needed to review her relationship to the **body**. Before this period, women cultivated a relationship of naturality and belonging, in which the body was a form of expression. From the rise of Christianity and the witch-hunt movement, the woman had to move ever further away from her body and closer to the soul through religion and charity[5].

With the creation of the first nursing schools at the end of the 19th century, care practices were fed by scientific knowledge, but they refused to deny the value of the body, for both the patient and the caregiver. The founder of modern nursing, **Florence Nightingale**, stated that, in order to care for others, nurses had to be able to first take care of themselves[5,10] so that they could approach the patient in an integrative way.

The concepts of health and care were developed from this moment on by **nursing** theories, considering the bio-psycho-social-spiritual context, integrality, interpersonal relationships, self-care and meeting health needs[11–13].

However, the **social perspective** of nursing regarding care has also suffered from a predominance of the biomedical model, leading to care that is focused on the physical and biological aspects, thus reducing the individuality of the patient and their social and community environment.

Fortunately, the **systemic view** of health has also prospered and influenced the development of social medicine and public health. Since 1700, the Italian Bernardino Ramazzini had already been associating working conditions with diseases, and in 1779, German Johan Peter Frank argued for the necessity of the State to take care of people's health[14,15]. This view was exacerbated by diseases arising from industrialization and the expansion of urban growth at different moments of public health[16], as characterized below:

1. **Empirical sanitation** (1840–1890): appreciated the cleanliness of air, water, and urban agglomerations.

2. **Bacteriological era** (until the first decade of the 20th century): based on the scientific application of bacteriology and the control of infectious diseases.

3. **Health education** (from the second decade of the 20th century): begins with the implementation of health centers that propose to take care of the community, in order to reach the individual through the collective.

The **"normal"** functioning of the body, which was equated to the proper functioning of a machine and recognized as synonymous with health, was expanded by the World Health Organization (WHO), who defined health as "a state of complete physical, mental and social well-being and not merely the absence of disease or infirmity"[17]. However, this same concept is questioned for being abstract and idealized[2], after all, we live with multiple expressions of illness and sickness that generate different perceptions of discomfort and suffering.

Some illnesses that are characterized as diseases are incorporated into our daily life, and do not always disqualify our **perception of health**. For example, if you have myopia, astigmatism or hyperopia, you have probably already adapted and incorporated the use of glasses or lenses into your routine, without compromising your well-being.

At the same time, natural changes throughout life, whether they are growth, aging, menstrual cycles, or physiological changes in pregnancy and menopause, make it difficult to maintain a complete state of well-being. The challenges, stresses and frustrations of everyday life also interfere with this utopian reference of **completeness**. The adoption of an idealized and unattainable condition is incompatible with practice and, by itself, can lead to illness by bringing the idea of health closer to perfection and moving it further away from the singularity with which it is expressed in our lives.

WHO, 40 years later, has broadened its vision of health by proposing a definition of **health promotion** in the Ottawa Charter[18]:

> "Health promotion is the process of enabling people to increase control over, and to improve, their health. To reach a state of complete physical, mental and social well-being, an individual or group must be able to identify and to realize aspirations, to satisfy needs, and to change or cope with the environment. Health is, therefore, seen as a resource for everyday life, not the objective of living. Health is a positive concept emphasizing social and personal resources, as well as physical capacities. Therefore, health promotion is not just the responsibility of the health sector, but goes beyond healthy lifestyles to well-being".

The promotion of health thus seeks to integrate technical and popular knowledge, based on an **expanded conception** of the health-disease process and its determinants that are related to the social and historical spheres of life and work, such as sanitation, housing, education, leisure, living habits, and economic, cultural and environmental conditions. According to this view, it invites professionals and patients to work together to address different health problems and needs[19].

Another effect of expanding the concept of health is to expand the choices of the individual, by encouraging **autonomy**, which calls for reflection and decision-making, so that the individual can exercise greater independence over their health[20].

From the second half of the 19th century on, different movements began to propose changes to the biomedical model. The **collective health** movement, which considers how the various health determinants influence each other, has opened up a new possibility for understanding the biopsychosocial complexity of the human being[21].

Together, the Latin American **sanitarist movement** and, particularly in Brazil, with its wave of health reforms proposed that health and disease depend on socioeconomic conditions such as income, employment, labor, and also on culture and values, including notions about sexuality, gender, among others[22].

By understanding the patient in their **uniqueness,** collective health seeks to assist them individually, fully and with respect, while recognizing their social and economic place as part of the community and social network that gives support in their life[23].

New **approaches** have been proposed to better respond to health-disease needs, such as the amplified clinical practice, humanization of care, integrality of actions and greater acceptance of alternative medicines[8]. Professionals who maintain contact with these approaches demonstrate broadened conceptions, that include the search for quality of life from a bio-psycho-socio-spiritual perspective[24].

Humanization of Care

In Brazil, the conception that guides public policies in the Unified Health System (Sistema Único de Saúde – SUS) presents health as a state of balance between the physical, psychological, social and cultural dimensions[25]. The National Policy of Humanization — **HumanizaSUS** — is guided by the values of autonomy, protagonism, co-responsibility among people, the establishment of solidarity bonds, the construction of cooperation networks and collective participation in the management process. It is based on nine "technologies" or "ways of doing" as described below[26]:

1. **Amplified clinic.** A clinical approach that aims to produce health and increase the autonomy of the person, the family and the community by increasing accessible resources. It uses as a means of working the integration of the multidisciplinary team, accountability, the construction of bonds and development of a Singular Therapeutic Project.

2. **Autonomy.** In its etymological sense, it means "the production of its own laws" or "the ability to abide by its own laws." To think of people as autonomous is to consider them protagonists and co-responsible for the health production process.

3. **Bond.** The encounter between patient and health worker promotes a meeting between two human beings, with their intentions, interpretations, needs, reasons and feelings, but in a situation of imbalance, with different abilities and expectations, in which one, the patient, seeks assistance, in a weakened physical and emotional state, together with the other, a professional supposedly qualified to attend and care for the cause of their fragility. This creates a bond, that is, an affective and moral connection between both, in a coexistence of mutual help and respect.

4. **Embracement.** The welcoming of the patient, upon arrival, occurs by taking full responsibility for them, listening to their complaints, allowing them to express their concerns, anxieties, and, at the same time, setting the necessary limits, ensuring resolute attention and articulation, when necessary, along with other health services essential for continuous care.

5. **Equality.** Access to actions and services, for the promotion, protection and recovery of health, is guaranteed through social

and economic policies aimed at reducing the risk of diseases and illnesses.

6. **Humanization.** Understood from an ethical-aesthetic-political approach, ethics implies a committed and co-responsible attitude of patients, managers and health workers; the aesthetics propose a creative and sensitive process for the production of health and the political aspect refers to the social and institutional organization of healthcare and management practices in the SUS network.

7. **Integrality.** The right of access to all spheres of health care, based on the establishment of a network of services acting with integrated actions, capable of providing integrative health care. The proposal of the integrative approach considers people in their inseparable biopsychosocial dimensions, overcoming the fragmentation of interventions.

8. **Protagonism.** The action, dialogue and attitude of people are central to the production of their own health.

9. **Universality.** It defines the State's duty to provide coverage, access to SUS and universal service in a fair and integral manner.

In this proposal, professionals and patients are responsible for the **co-development** of care by exchanging, signs and symptoms, but also facts, emotions and feelings, in a dynamic and progressive process, in which "care is about meeting another person to accompany them in the promotion of their health, from the creation, cultivation and maintenance of bonds of trust and connection"[27:201][Translation].

Efforts to expand the concepts of health and care, however, demand social and collective transformations to reach people, both professionals and patients, training centers and health services, and generate conceptions compatible with this vision. Would it be a **utopia**? Perhaps, but we need to aim for the horizon if we want to get closer to it.

The different conceptions of health and care require **changes** in the work process that expresses the practice and dynamics of work exercised by health professionals, such as the time of care, the way in which professionals interact with patients and the relationship between the work team[28].

They also require new **approaches** to accompany these changes, in order to modify the work models adopted, integrate other technologies and "ways of doing things", incorporate integrative and complementary therapies, dialogue with other paradigms, and expand the production of knowledge in health.

Each concept of health expresses different **worldviews** that profoundly impact the care practices offered. Therefore, understanding the complexity of health concepts is essential for improving health and care in a variety of contexts[29].

In fact, individuals and societies consider themselves to be more or less healthy, depending on the moment, the framework and the values they attribute to a situation. Thus, it is possible to say that an understanding of health and care merge aspects of subjectivity and **historical-social determinants**. Health cannot be seen as something alien to people, because everything that is said about health is said by someone and for someone[30], while it is not separated from cultural interpretations, since people are part of social collectives.

This brief **overview** of the evolution of the concepts of health and care from antiquity through to modern social, preventive, public and collective health, recovers relevant moments in the generation of knowledge and health practices. In this respect, it intends to support the reading of the next chapters, without the intention of exhausting this subject, which is constantly changing.

What **concept of health** do you *express* in everyday life? As a health professional, what concept of health is perceived in the way you work? How do concepts of health *influence* your **self-care**?

Chapter 2
Integrative Health

Paracelsus (1493–1541)

Have you heard about *integrative health*? When you think of
complementary therapies, what comes to your mind? The purpose of this chapter is to present different health and care practices
based on different **rationales**.

In the second half of the 20th century, there was a strong pressure from **social movements** in search of sustainable development
and improved quality of life, that sought to recover the individual's
natural capacity to promote their own health, with an appreciation
of traditional, alternative and complementary practices[6].

The growing demand for **alternative practices** was concomitant with the increasing difficulties faced by Western medicine and its inability to focus on the person and their care shared between patients and health professionals[9]. In complementary therapies, the object of care is not the disease, but the individual in a state of imbalance, to be guided and assisted in restoring or expanding their health[31].

Alternative practices are focused on the person's life **experience**, particularly with an emphasis on the patient, not the disease. Such practices have an integrative, non-interventionist, holistic, systemic and interdisciplinary character. In general, they criticize biological reductionism, mechanicism and the predominance of the disease over the patient that characterizes modern medicine[7].

From this perspective, sociologist Madel Luz developed the concept of **medical rationales**, understood as complex medical systems composed of six structural dimensions, which coexist and interact in contemporary culture[32]. She carried out comparative studies of four rationales: contemporary Western medicine or biomedicine; homeopathy; traditional Chinese medicine and ayurvedic medicine. The six structural dimensions are[33]:

1. **Cosmology:** presents the fundamental basis and explains the relationship of individuals, families, society and the universe.

2. **Medical doctrine:** conceptualizes health, disease, treatment and the cure.

3. **Morphology:** it shows the anatomy, considering organs, viscera, tissue constitution, vital force, energetic meridians.

4. **Physiology or vital dynamics:** presents the functioning of systems, illness, medicines and the energetic dimension.

5. **Diagnosis:** presents the diagnostic system, based on the identification of imbalances, symptoms, physical examination and complementary examinations.

6. **Therapy:** presents treatments and care related to hygiene, food, medicine, massages, among others.

The contribution of medical rationales consists in creating parameters that allow us to see other medical systems as carriers of **scientific rationality** and to distinguish between what are medical systems and therapeutic practices, also called health practices. And, consequently, they contribute to the institutional legitimacy of these medical systems in health policies, recognizing them as bearers of theoretical coherence and therapeutic consistency that support their application[33].

Since 1978, **WHO** has proposed the use of alternative therapeutic practices, not institutionalized by the health system, as important measures to improve the health of the community[7]. To this end, it promotes the safety, quality and efficiency of these practices and encourages the formulation and implementation of public policies and national regulations. Thus, inclusion encourages planning for the integration of traditional and complementary/alternative medicine into the already offered health service, considering the products and practices offered and the recognition of its practitioners[34–36].

Traditional medicine demarcates the set of knowledge and practices, based on theories, beliefs and the experiences of different cultures, whether they are explained or not, used to maintain health and prevent, diagnose and treat diseases. The concepts of **complementary or alternative medicine** define a broad set of health practices that are not part of a country's tradition or conventional medicine, nor are they fully integrated into the prevailing health system. In some countries, the concepts of complementary or alternative medicine may also refer to traditional medicine[37].

The World Health Organization **Atlas** on the use of traditional and complementary/alternative medicine[38] found that 88% of its member countries recognize and use these practices. The nine most used are:

1. Acupuncture.

2. Ayurvedic medicine.

3. Chiropractic.

4. Phytotherapy.

5. Homeopathy.

6. Naturopathy.

7. Osteopathy.

8. Traditional Chinese medicine.

9. Unani medicine.

Another **research study**[39] identified the use of these practices in the general population and among health professionals in ten countries, without including Brazil. The results indicated that the most used practices, in decreasing order excluding the practice of prayer, were chiropractic, phytotherapy, massage and homeopathy. The practices found were grouped under these five categories:

1. **Medical systems:** acupuncture, ayurveda, homeopathy, naturopathy, traditional Chinese medicine.

2. **Biological therapies:** aromatherapy, chelation, dietary therapies, folk medicine, iridology, megavitamin therapy, neural therapy, phytotherapy.

3. **Energy medicine:** healing, light therapy, magnetotherapy, millimiter wave therapy, reiki, sound energy therapy.

4. **Manual therapies:** acupressure, Alexander technique, Bowen technique, chiropractic, Feldrenkrais method, massage, osteopathy, reflexology, Rolfing, Trager bodywork, tuina.

5. **Mind-Body therapies:** anthroposophic medicine, autogenic training, biofeedback, bioresonance, cognitive-behavioral therapy, deep breathing exercises, group support, hypnosis, imagery, meditation, prayer, relaxation, qi gong, tai chi, yoga, shiatsu, spiritual healing.

This research also identified the **diseases** most frequently associated with the use of complementary and alternative medicines, which included back pain or disease, depression, insomnia, severe headaches or migraines, and stomach or intestinal diseases[39].

Integrative and Complementary Practices

In **Brazil**, the inclusion of these practices in the Unified Health System (SUS) is guided by the National Policy of Integrative and Complementary Practices (Política Nacional de Práticas Integrativas e Complementares – PNPIC), based on the vision of continued, humanized and integrative health care[25]. PNPIC includes alternative and complementary medicines and the appreciation of traditional practices and popular wisdom. The proposal is to offer different practices with the purpose of recovering the individual's responsibility for their own health, while questioning the surrender of a person's health care to the pharmaceutical and hospital industry[7].

The **PNPIC**, published in 2006, initially included five health care practices, which are presented below[25]:

1. **Anthroposophical medicine.** It is a complementary, vitalist-based medical-therapeutic approach, whose care model is organized in a transdisciplinary manner, with the participation of physicians and other health professionals. It uses drugs specific to anthroposophic medicine, as well as homeopathic and herbal medicines.

2. **Homeopathy.** A complex, holistic medical system, based on the vitalist principle and the law of similars enunciated by Hippocrates in the 4th century BCE. It was developed by Samuel Hahnemann in the 18th century. The law of similars (*Similia si-*

milibus curantur) states that a substance capable of causing certain harmful effects in an organism can also cure similar effects in a sick organism. It uses homeopathic medicines.

3. **Medicinal plants and Phytotherapy.** Therapy characterized by the use of medicinal plants in their different pharmaceutical forms, without the use of isolated active substances, although of plant origin. The use of medicinal plants as a form of treatment has very ancient origins, relating to the beginnings of society.

4. **Thermalism — Crenotherapy.** The use of mineral waters for health treatment dates from the time of the Greek Empire, as described by Herodotus in 450 BCE. Thermalism involves the different ways of using mineral water in health treatments or for preservation. Crenotherapy is the indication and use of mineral waters for therapeutic purposes, as a complement to other health treatments.

5. **Traditional Chinese medicine — Acupuncture.** A complete medical system, that originated thousands of years ago in China. It uses language that symbolically portrays the laws of nature and values the harmonious interrelation between the parties aiming at their integrity. As a foundation, it points out the theory of Yin-yang and that of the five movements: wood, fire, earth, metal and water. For diagnosis, it uses a medical history, palpation of the wrist, and observation of the face and tongue. It applies several treatment modalities, such as acupuncture, auriculotherapy, medicinal plants, diet therapy, body and mental practices.

PNPIC recognizes that these practices have the **stimulus** of natural mechanisms in common for the prevention of illness and disease and promote health through effective, safe technologies, through an emphasis on receptive listening, development of the therapeutic bond and integration of the human being into the environment and society[25].

Reducing **costs** through the provision of complementary therapies is also a motivator for its incorporation into health systems, however, it should not be understood as a goal, but as a result. The cost of homeopathic intervention and traditional Chinese medicine is very low compared to the interventions of Western medicine, mainly because it guarantees a broad therapeutic process, which emancipates people and lowers the risk of iatrogenic conditions, that result from adverse effects or complications of treatment[40].

The **offer** of complementary therapies in the SUS increases each year, reaching 54% of Brazilian municipalities and 100% of the capitals in 2018[41]. At the same time, supply has grown in the private sector. However, there are still many challenges for policy implementation in the SUS network, and this is an on-going process.

In 2017, the Ministry of Health expanded **access** to fourteen more practices by including them in the PNPIC[42]:

1. **Art therapy.** It uses art as the basis of the therapeutic process, through painting, drawing, sounds, music, modeling, collage, mime, weaving, body expression, sculpturing, among others. It can be performed individually or in a group. Art therapy is based on the principle that the creative process is therapeutic and enhances one's quality of life. It seeks to bring new meaning to conflicts, reorganizes the individual's own perceptions and broadens their perception of themselves and the world.

2. **Ayurveda.** Developed in India during the period 2000–1000 BCE, ayurveda means the Science or Knowledge of life. It combines principles related to the health of the physical body con-

sidering the energetic, mental and spiritual fields, and the theory of the three *doshas* (biological humors). Each *dosha* is related to a subtle essence: *Vata*, to vital energy; *Pitta*, to essential fire; and *Kapha*, to mental energy. The diagnostic investigation considers the affected site and body tissues, the *doshas*, resistance and vitality, daily routine, eating habits, digestive condition, personal and social details, and the economic and environmental situation of the person. Relaxation techniques, massages, medicinal plants, minerals, *asanas* (body postures), *pranayamas* (respiratory techniques), *mudras* (positions and exercises) and dietary care are used.

3. **Biodance.** It is a systemic approach based on the most primitive origins of dance, that seeks to reestablish the individual's connection with themselves, with others and with the environment. Its methodology consists in inducing integrative collective experiences, in an environment enriched with selected stimuli such as music, songs, exercises and activities capable of generating experiences that stimulate neuronal plasticity and the creation of new synaptic networks. In this sense, biodance is configured as a system for accelerating the existential integrative processes: psychological, neurological, endocrinological and immunological, studied by Psycho-Neuro-Endocrine-Immunology (PNEI), producing health effects by activating the whole organism and generating adaptive and integrative processes, through optimizing the organism's homeostasis.

4. **Circular dancing.** Sacred Circle Dancing or simply Circle Dancing is a traditional and contemporary, circular dance practice, originating from different cultures, that favor learning and the harmonious interconnection between participants. Through the rhythm, melody and delicate and deep movements, members of the circle are encouraged to respect, accept and honor diversity. In the circle, the balance between the individual and the collective, the feeling of belonging and pleasure for full participation in internal

transformation processes, promote well-being, harmony between body-mind-spirit, the elevation of self-esteem, body awareness, and other benefits.

5. **Chiropractic.** A care practice that uses manipulative diagnostic and therapeutic elements, aimed at the treatment and prevention of neuro-musculoskeletal system disorders and their effects on health in general. The chiropractor uses his hands to apply controlled force to the joint, pressing beyond the usual range of motion. The promoted joint adjustment aims to influence joint and neurophysiological functions to correct the subluxation complex, described as a segmental motor dysfunction, composed by the interaction of pathological changes in nervous, muscular, ligamentous, vascular and connective tissues.

6. **Integrative Community Therapy (ICT).** It is an intervention practice in social groups that aims to create and strengthen social solidarity networks. It leverages the resources of the community and is based on the principle that the community and its individuals have problems, but they can also develop resources, skills and strategies to solve difficulties. It is an area which welcomes psychic suffering by favoring the exchange of experiences between people. ICT is developed in a wheel format, designed to work on the horizontal and circular levels. Each participant in the session is co-responsible for the therapeutic process, producing individual and collective effects. The sharing of experiences aims at valuing personal stories, thus favoring the recovery of identity, the restoration of self-esteem and self-confidence, the expansion of perception and the possibility of solving problems.

7. **Meditation.** It is a practice of harmonizing mental states and awareness, present in many cultures and traditions. Meditation makes the person attentive, through experiencing what the mind is

doing in the present moment, and developing self-knowledge and awareness, in order to observe one's thoughts and reduce their flow. It is an instrument of physical, emotional, mental, social and cognitive strengthening. The practice benefits the cognitive system, promotes concentration, helps one to perceive physical and emotional sensations, thus increasing one's self-discipline in health care. Additionally, it stimulates well-being and relaxation, and reduces stress, hyperactivity and depressive symptoms.

8. **Music therapy.** It is the use of music and its elements (sound, rhythm, melody and harmony), in a group or in an individualized way, to facilitate and promote communication, relationship-building, learning, mobilization, expression, organization and other relevant therapeutic goals, in order to satisfy physical, emotional, mental, social and cognitive needs. It aims to develop potential and reestablish individual functions so that one can achieve better intra and interpersonal integration and, consequently, a better quality of life. It favors creative, emotional and affective development while physically activating touch, hearing, breathing, circulation and the reflexes.

9. **Naturopathy.** It is understood as a care practice that, through natural methods and resources, supports and stimulates the intrinsic capacity of the body to heal itself. Its origin is based on the health-care knowledge of diverse cultures, particularly those that consider vitalism, a vital principle existing in each individual which influences the organic, emotional and mental balance of their worldview. It uses various therapeutic resources, such as medicinal plants, mineral and thermal waters, aromatherapy, trophology, massage, expressive resources, mind-body therapies and changes of habit.

10. **Osteopathy.** It is a diagnostic and therapeutic method that works on the individual, in an integral way, based on the ma-

nipulation of joints and tissues. This practice assumes that joint and tissue mobility disorders generally contribute to the appearance of diseases. The osteopathic approach involves deep anatomical, physiological and global biomechanical knowledge, relating all systems to formulate diagnostic hypotheses and apply the treatments effectively. Thus, osteopathy differs from other manipulation methods, as it seeks to work in an integral way, providing conditions for the organism to seek balance and homeostasis.

11. **Reiki.** It is a practice of laying hands that involves coming close to or touching the person's body to stimulate the natural mechanisms of health recovery. Based on the vitalist conception of health, it considers the existence of a channeled universal energy that acts on the balance of vital energy for the purpose of harmonizing the general conditions of the body and mind. The therapy aims to strengthen the places where there are blockages (energetic nodes), eliminating toxins and balancing full cellular functioning to restore the flow of vital energy. The practice promotes harmonization between the physical, mental and spiritual dimensions. It stimulates the energizing of organs and energetic centers. The practice of Reiki considers the dimensions of the consciousness, body, emotions, activates the glands, organs, nervous, cardiac and immune system. Additionally, it assists in the treatment of stress, depression and anxiety, and promotes the balance of vital energy.

12. **Reflexotherapy.** It is a practice that uses stimuli in reflex areas for therapeutic purposes. It assumes that the body is crossed by meridians that divide it into different regions. Each of these regions has its own reflex zone, especially on the feet or in the hands. Key points are massaged that enable the reactivation of homeostasis and the balance of body regions where some kind of blockage or inconvenience occurs. Areas of the body are projected onto the feet, hands, ears and other body regions, and are known as microsystems or reflex areas.

13. **Shantala.** It is a massage practice for babies and children, composed of a series of bodily movements that promotes the awakening and expanding of the bond between the caregiver and baby. Thus, it fosters and strengthens the affective bond, cooperation, trust, creativity, security, physical and emotional balance, and promotes integral health. It enables the baby and the child to stimulate their joints and muscles, significantly assisting in motor development, facilitating movements such as rolling, sitting, crawling and walking.

14. **Yoga.** It is a practice that combines physical postures, breathing techniques, meditation and relaxation. It strengthens the musculoskeletal system, stimulates the endocrine system, expands respiratory capacity and exercises the cognitive system. It uses *asana* (body postures), *pranayamas* (respiratory techniques) and *mudras* (positions and exercises). It also advocates self-care, healthy eating and the practice of nonviolent ethics. Its practice improves quality of life, reduces stress, decreases heart rate and blood pressure, relieves anxiety, depression and insomnia, and improves physical fitness, strength and overall flexibility.

In March 2018, the Ministry of Health held the I International Congress of Integrative practices and Public Health (**Intercongrepics**), which valued complementary therapies at a national and international level. During the event, ten new practices were included in PNPIC, namely[43,44]:

1. **Apitherapy.** A therapeutic practice that consists of using products derived from bees such as apitoxins, honey, pollen, royal jelly and propolis, for promoting health and therapeutic purposes.

2. **Aromatherapy.** A therapeutic practice that uses the properties of essential oils to recover the balance and harmony of the organism in order to promote physical and mental health.

3. **Bioenergetic.** A practice that adopts body psychotherapy and therapeutic exercises in groups to release the body's tension and facilitate the expression of feelings.

4. **Chromotherapy.** A therapeutic practice using the colors of the solar spectrum — red, orange, yellow, green, blue, indigo and violet — to restore the physical and energetic balance of the body.

5. **Family constellation.** A psychotherapeutic method that seeks, through knowledge of the forces that act in the family unconscious and the laws of human relationships, to find order, belonging and balance, while creating conditions for the person to reorient their movement towards healing and growth. It is a therapy that was developed in the 80's by the German psychotherapist Bert Hellinger, which can be done in groups, during workshops, or in individual sessions.

6. **Flower therapy.** A therapeutic practice that uses essences derived from flowers to modify certain vibratory states, helping to balance and harmonize the individual. Created by the Englishman Dr. Edward Bach (1886–1936), Bach's floral therapy is a pioneering system, which then diversified into other floral systems, such as the Australian, Californian, Minas, Saint Germain, Cerrado, Joel Aleixo, Mystica, Alaska and Hawaii systems.

7. **Geotherapy.** A natural therapeutic practice that consists in the use of medical clay, mud and sludge, with the objective of caring for physical and emotional imbalances through the different types of energy and chemical properties of these elements. Geotherapy rebalances the energetic and meridian centers of the body, facilitates contact with the inner self and works therapeutically with the reflex zones.

8. **Hypnotherapy.** A set of techniques that, by means of intense relaxation, concentration and/or focus, induce the person to achieve an increased state of awareness that allows for the changing

of a wide range of undesirable conditions or behaviors, such as fears, phobias, insomnia, depression, anxiety, stress and chronic pain.

9. **Imposition of hands.** A secular therapeutic practice that involves the laying on of hands and a meditative effort for the transfer of vital energy (*Qi, prana*) through the hands as a way to restore the balance of the human energetic field, thus assisting in the health-disease process.

10. **Ozone therapy.** It uses a mixture of oxygen and ozone gases, through different routes of administration, and has a therapeutic purpose of improving several diseases.

In addition to the 29 complementary therapies, other practices have also been developed by health professionals to expand integrative care and promote health. The Thematic **Glossary** of Integrative and Complementary Practices presents more than 110 practices reflecting different medical rationales[44].

The proposition and incorporation of new complementary therapies and health approaches is **dynamic**, follows scientific development, and can be exemplified by the ten methods and movements described below, which have emerged in recent decades:

1. **Eutonia**[b]. A somatic educational approach created by the German Gerda Alexander (1908–1994), which uses the observation and reception of physical sensations and body postures, with the objective of promoting an expansion of perception and body awareness that contributes to the care of pain and stress and improves the adaptability of the body to everyday life[45].

2. **Microphysiotherapy**[c]. A manual therapy technique developed in France during the early 80s, by physiotherapists and oste-

---

b https://eutoni.dk/
c http://microkinesitherapie.fr/en/microphysiotherapy/

opaths Drs. Daniel Grosjean and Patrice Benine. The therapy works with a body map, through specific and gentle manual gestures with the objective of releasing scars that interfere with tissue functioning and alter its vital rhythm, thus promoting the balance and maintenance of health.

3. **McKenzie method**[d]. A method of evaluation and treatment of pain in the spine, neck and extremities, developed by the New Zealand physiotherapist Robin McKenzie, in the 50's. It combines postural orientation and the individualized application of specific exercises prescribed by the professional, which enables the patient to individually treat their condition and prevent recurrences.

4. **Mindfulness.** A practice that focuses on the experience of accepting the present as it is. This implies breaking out of the usual standards of judgment and criticism and adopting a curious and kind attitude towards the experience, that changes how the inevitable difficulties of life affect the person. It was popularized by Jon Kabat-Zinn in the 70s, who applied the Buddhist concept of full attention, but removed any religious aspect from the practice[46]. Scientific evidence[e] shows numerous positive effects of mindfulness and meditation, such as reducing stress and pain and improving one's quality of life. Apps and websites, such as *Headspace*[f] and *Zen*[g], provide tools that make it easier to develop the person's practice. Different centers in Brazil, such as the Unifesp Mente Aberta Mindfulness Brasil[h], apply and study specific protocols of mindfulness focused on promoting health, compassion, mindful eating or for specifically treating stress, depression and chemical dependence.

---

d   https://mckenzieinstitute.org/
e   https://mtci.bvsalud.org/en/clinical-effectiveness-of-meditation/
f   https://www.headspace.com/
g   zen-guided-meditation-sleep/id1089982285
h   https://mindfulnessbrasil.com/

5. **Positive psychology.** A psychology movement that started in 1998 by Martin Seligman, along with Mihaly Csikszentmihalyi, Christopher Peterson and Barbara Fredrickson. It is dedicated to the study of positive human functioning and development (flourishing), as opposed to the focus of psychology on mental disease. In the book Positivity[47], the author Barbara Fredrickson presents tools to live better as well as strategies to reduce negativity. Among them is the positivity quotient of 3 to 1, that is, evidence demonstrates the need for three positive factors to overcome a negative factor. Achieving this ratio is not an easy task, so tools were developed to measure this process, available on their website[i]. Positivity is also the subject of research by various renowned authors in books such as Flourish[48], The Happiness Advantage[49] and Positive Intelligence[50].

6. **Lifestyle medicine[j].** An interdisciplinary approach developed from the 2000's that prioritizes the therapeutic use of lifestyle to help individuals and families adopt and maintain healthy behaviors that affect their health and quality of life, such as nutrition, physical activity, sleep, stress management, healthy relationships, in addition to other non-medicated modalities.

7. **Slow medicine[k].** A movement which started in Italy in the 2000's that seeks to recover the time and attention dedicated by the professional to the patient, enabling the patient to carefully assess and understand their broader health context, while avoiding hasty diagnoses and unnecessary treatments and contributing to their cure.

8. **Spiral taping.** A therapy developed in the 80's by the Japanese acupuncturist and osteopath, Nobutaka Tanaka, for the treatment of pain associated with orthopedic and rheumatic problems. It

---

i   positivityratio.com
j   https://www.lifestylemedicine.org/
k   https://www.slowmedicine.it/

uses the bonding of spiral-shaped adhesive tapes, that are drug-free and non-immobilizing, for the treatment of edemas and muscle and joint pain, with the objective of restoring the body's general balance[51].

9. **Neurofeedback.** An operant conditioning modality that trains with the use of devices that monitor brain conditions, with the objective of restoring the appropriate patterns of brain functioning. It is used for the treatment of neurological, psychiatric or psychological disorders, for the promotion of cognitive abilities, an increase in personal performance and a feeling of well-being. Neurofeedback's use for the treatment of attention deficit is scientifically established and it's developing use for non-clinical conditions continues[52].

10. **EMDR** (*Eye Movement Desensitization and Reprocessing*): a psychotherapeutic method that uses bilateral sensory stimuli, such as horizontal eye movements from side to side, manual touches or vibrational stimuli interspersing the right and left sides of the body. Developed by Francine Shapiro in the 1990's, the method aims to reduce suffering and strengthen adaptive beliefs related to trauma.

In the book **The Instinct to Heal**, Dr. David Servan-Schreiber[53] presents therapies for treating stress, anxiety and depression, such as respiratory and communication techniques, physical exercises, exposure to light, cardiac consistency, intake of omega 3, acupuncture and EMDR. According to the researcher, these practices can broaden the therapeutic approach by directly influencing the emotional brain through the body, without using the path of language and reasoning, that often characterize the cognitive brain.

In this evolving context of complementary therapies, the concept of **integrative health** continues to develop. Built from an expansion of the concept of integrative medicine[54], it consists of six aspects listed below:

1. Integration of alternative and complementary medicine with conventional medicine.

2. Combining ancient healing systems with modern Western medicine.

3. Valuing the physician-patient relationship and communication.

4. Consideration of the person as a whole.

5. Use of scientific evidence.

6. Focus on health, healing and disease prevention.

Integrative health invites us to **rethink** the type of relationship established by the person with themselves, with the health service and professionals, in addition to the relationship between the health professionals. Therefore, it does not propose replacing existing practices, for example, by suspending the use of medication, to insert acupuncture needles, or to use phytotherapy in its place, but, rather, to act in an integrated manner, from a new perspective.

However, **curative hegemony** within the health care environment and professional training centers has made it difficult to incorporate complementary therapies into health services[9], because these practices change health and structural care concepts of the biomedical model. This hegemony also prevents the spread of the idea that there is no ideal care, but an exchange of knowledge among those involved in the process in which they, together, make the best decision[27].

A barrier to be overcome for the integration of complementary therapies is the lack of knowledge concerning the practice itself and the available scientific **evidence**[24]. Therefore, in 2018, the Virtual Health Library (VHL) in Traditional, Complementary and Integrative Medicines (TCIM) was created. This is a thematic and specialized library, which promotes open access to information and facilitates the visibility of experiences and good practices in TCIM[1].

Evidence is critical to promote the use and discussion of and also draw action limits for each practice, especially when considering these three **myths**:

1. **Complementary therapies are harmless.** Any therapeutic action has the potential to produce undesirable or adverse effects. Some herbal medicines, for example, may interact with other medications in use by the patient, altering the original result of these substances; manual therapies, such as massage, may initially aggravate the muscular pain felt by the patient before producing the desired relief. When we work with health, it is more prophylactic to adopt the principle that there is no innocuous therapy. Therefore, it is essential that professionals and patients always talk about the use, application and effects of these practices.

2. **Complementary therapies have a placebo effect.** The placebo response occurs when the patient has positive results when subjected to supposedly unspecific and apparently inert factors, such as a verbal or visual suggestion, taking a pill without any active substance (sugar or flour), injection of a saline solution or sham surgery. Typically, the placebo effect affects up to one third of patients participating in scientific studies, and is attributed to the symbolism that the treatment exercises as a result of the patient's positive expectation. Its opposite is the *nocebo effect*, when the results generated are negative. However, some researchers have investigated the power of conviction and positive expectation to change the brain's neurochemical pattern, elevating the placebo to a therapy capable of recovering and transforming the organism, with psychoneurophysiologi-

1 https://mtci.bvsalud.org/en/

cal bases[55]. This phenomenon, commonly related to complementary therapies, can also be enhanced by incorporating human aspects of care into the relationship between professionals and patients.

3. **Complementary therapies don't work for serious diseases.** Faced with a heart attack, fractured arm or lymphoma, the most reasonable therapeutic option adopted will be Western medicine. However, since antiquity, many practices have been developed to treat these diseases, especially when current medical resources did not yet exist. The South Korean sitcom *Live up to your name* (*Myeongbulheojeon*, 2017) explores this conflict of adopting traditional Korean medicine practices in modern times to treat serious conditions, even though they may be as effective as modern ones. Without taking the place of the main therapy, there are still many indications for complementary therapies in these cases, because, by interacting and acting in synergy with other treatments, they help augment the well-being and results achieved, as viewed from an integral health perspective.

Most patients do not report or talk about which complementary therapies they use with their physicians for fear of judgment and rebuke, which can increase the risk for the treatments performed and the discontinuity of these practices[56]. In addition to the discredit of some health professionals, who do not usually apply the same criteria in the analysis of allopathic treatments and their risks, complementary therapies also face **difficulties** in producing scientific evidence relating to the biomedical approach. In part, they are limitations resulting from the research model, whose positivist and quantitative basis opposes the subjectivity and integrative approach of these practices. Another added obstacle is the lack of financial resources, as it is rare that pharmaceutical industries and research funding agencies are interested in investing in producing research related to such practices.

The dissemination of complementary therapies and its results proposes a more humane and integral care **path**, improving the ability to respond to the needs of the individual and the community. On the one hand, despite the advances, the low supply and difficulties in referring patients to these practices are obstacles resulting from the characteristics of biomedical knowledge, which are present in the training of professionals, as well as in the performance of health services.

On the other hand, specific training **courses** in complementary therapies offered by SUS are increasing, as well as online courses in Auriculotherapy promoted by the Federal University of Santa Catarina (UFSC) and the Residency Program in Integrative and Complementary Practices in Primary Health Care offered by the Municipal Health Department of São Paulo. This also includes courses promoted through private initiatives, such as the Graduate Course in Integrative Health and Wellness offered by the Israeli Albert Einstein Institute of Teaching and Research.

However, the variety and heterogeneity of the **training** courses available in complementary therapies have raised questions about their duration, quality and high cost[24]. In addition to training, another growing discussion concerns the minimum curriculum requirements of professionals who can offer these therapies in the public and private health systems. The professional councils and the associations of practitioners have been developing this discussion, yet are still far from a consensus.

Moreover, the **private market** for complementary therapy services, present in Brazil and in countries such as Australia, the

United States, Canada and Germany, is of concern to profession-als[24], since it places these practices as a deluxe service, that is, accessible only to those who can afford them. Thus, it is important that public health systems avoid a deeply delegitimizing equation: allowing therapeutic plurality (or access to complementary therapies) for the rich, while the poor are left with the rigor (and limits) of conventional medicine[40].

Faced with a heterogeneous and under construction scenario, it is essential to broaden our understanding of complementary therapies and integrative health, especially when considering its benefits, risks and possibilities of integration with Western medicine. This path allows for the redefinition of health and care concepts, to meet the needs of each person, based on a **strategy** to develop their autonomy and qualify the bond with health professionals.

What is your level of **openness** to knowing and experiencing *new* *health and care* **practices**? Do you develop ***integrated therapeutic plans***, that contemplate more than one type of health practice?

Chapter 3
Consciential Health

"Conventional scientists fight against parapsychism because it is a force that escapes them. For centuries they have been imitating the fable of the fox and the grapes."

Waldo Vieira (1932–2015)[1:377][Translation]

Are you aware of the **interactions** between different *environments, energies, thoughts,* and the quality of your health? And between your *health* and your ***life projects and life purpose***? The objectives of this chapter are to broaden the understanding of health and care from a *multidimensional perspective* and to present the **principles of consciential health**.

Since antiquity, magical-religious conceptions of health and disease have admitted the influence of **supernatural forces** acting in the organism, often resulting from faith, sins or curses[4]. This conception of health is still present and observed in the popular culture of healing, shamanism, blessings, prayers, magic, spells and potions.

Some conceptions emphasize the harmony of human beings with themselves and with **nature**. The writings attributed to Hippocrates (460–370 BCE)[57] strengthen, in this sense, the connection between bodies, stars and nature and understand health as being the balance of the different dimensions of the individual, both physical and spiritual[58]. They oppose the sacred origin of diseases, reconciling human nature with the divine:

> "And the disease called the sacred arises from causes as the others, namely, those things which enter and quit the body, such as cold, the sun, and the winds, which are ever changing and are never at rest. And these things are divine, so that there is no necessity for making a distinction, and holding this disease to be more divine than the others, but all are divine, and all human."[59].

Galen (129–c199/c217CE), a physician and philosopher in the Roman Empire, revisited the humoral **doctrine** applied by Hippocrates to medicine and stressed the importance of the four temperaments in the state of health, supported by the four humors of the human body: blood, phlegm, yellow bile and black bile. Galens's theory saw the cause of the disease as endogenous, that is, it would be within man himself, in his physical constitution or in life habits that lead to imbalance. The humoral doctrine predominated in medical practice for more than 2,000 years, beginning its decline at the end of the 18th century[60].

Another aspect considered influential in health since antiquity are the **emanations** from unhealthy regions capable of causing diseases, as mentioned in *Corpus Hippocraticus*[4] and corroborated by physician Ibn Sina, popularly known as Avicena (980–1037 CE). This theory suggested that any place with infected air, such as rotten water, caves and excrement, should be avoided, because the bad odors were known to be important in explaining the transmission of diseases[61].

The importance of the humoral doctrine and bad odors in medieval health is portrayed in the literary work *Regimen Sanitatis*

Salernitanum, produced by the **Salerno School of Medicine** in the 13th century, and which spread throughout Europe. Written in verse, it advises good habits, is preventive in nature, and gives guidance on food, sleep, hygiene, the avoidance of impregnated air and the characteristics of the body's humors.

In contrast to the traditional medical notions of his time, Descartes' studies (1596–1650) emerged, with profound reflections on the way that **science** and medicine was performed. In his work Discourse on Method (1637), Descartes presents the bases of his scientific vision, giving rise to modern rationalism. He also discusses medical knowledge, refusing to follow it without questioning the established knowledge of medical books written by recognized and traditional authorities[62].

In the following centuries, the **scientific revolution** further expanded rational discourse and freedom of thought. With this, new scientific perspectives emerged for the study of *supernatural forces* and their relationship to health. In the 18th century, Mesmer (1734–1815) proposed the existence of a *force*, a *universal fluid*, that could affect our bodies and directly impact our personal health. Called animal magnetism, this force allowed celestial bodies, terrestrial objects and living beings to interact, enabling reciprocal and dynamic exchanges, even from a distance.

Animal magnetism was said to have healing and restorative properties, which could be captured, stored and transmitted for therapeutic purposes. To be healthy was thus to be in harmony with the universal fluid. The application of this knowledge by the physician, in the words of Mesmer, makes the art of healing reach its ultimate perfection[58].

Mesmer was influenced by Vitalism, an enlightening thought that considered the existence of a **vital principle** in living beings, responsible for the maintenance of health and life, as opposed to the prevailing materialism. This principle was already defended by the Swiss physician and philosopher Paracelsus (1493–1541) in the 16th century, recognized for his innovations in medical treatments, and a pioneer in opposing the hegemonic humoral doctrine of the time[63,64].

In the 19th century, Charles Richet (1850–1935) described the existence of a substance exteriorized from the bodies of mediums, during the spiritist phenomena of materialization, which he called **ectoplasm**. Such substance has amorphous, gelatinous and volatile characteristics. This concept, however, is not investigated by Richet from a therapeutic perspective[58], even though in spiritism its application has been widespread, from the laying on of hands to surgeries performed by mediums, in search of spiritual healing.

The various conceptions of health and disease pointed out so far reveal, each in its own time, different views of the world that qualify what is admitted as **real**. Likewise, to understand what conscientical health is, and under what precepts and worldview it was built on, it is important to understand what conscientiology is.

Conscientiology

Conscientiology is the science applied to the study of the **consciousness**, recognized as being, self, ego or intelligent principle, perceived in an integral, multidimensional, multiexistential and holosomatic way[65]. Proposed and founded by the Brazilian researcher Waldo Vieira (1932–2015), at the end of the 20th century,[66] it was initially developed in Brazil and today has volunteer researchers worldwide.

The **consciential paradigm**, which underlies its ideas, acts in contrast to conventional modern science. According to Vieira, conventional science accommodates itself to the physicalist perspective, avoiding the direct research of the object of consciousness in its approach, in a contradictory or irrational manner[67:22]. The consciential paradigm, on the other hand, aims to understand the reality of the consciousness on a broader level, considering at least ten conditions presented below:

1. **Consciousness:** in the universe there are two realities: *consciousnesses* and *energies*. The consciousness is the being, ego, self, the vital or intelligent principle, in continuous evolution. Energies are forces or substances lacking intelligence and their own will in different states of density. The consciousness uses energies to manifest themselves, imprinting on them their personal pattern, and mobilizing them by their own will.

2. **Multidimensionality:** the consciousness manifests themselves in multiple existential dimensions that coexist and interpenetrate one other. The *intraphysical dimension* is the physical, material, or human dimension where we typically manifest ourselves with the physical body. The *extraphysical dimensions* are non-physical dimensions, of a more subtle nature, and are popularly known as astral or spiritual plans. There are numerous gradations of extraphysical dimensions, from the most harmonious to the most disharmonious, with different levels of organization and *extraphysical communities* installed in these environments.

3. **Holosomatics:** the consciousness has four bodies or *vehicles of manifestation*, which overlap and intertwine with one another: soma, energosoma, psychosoma and mentalsoma. The *soma* is the biological, material and physical body. It is renewed at each rebirth, and discarded at the end of each life by biological death. The *energosoma* is the vitalizing energetic vehicle, also called the energetic body or holochakra. The *psychosoma* is the body of emotions, also

known as the perispirit, or spiritual body. The *mentalsoma* is the vehicle of discernment and ideas. The four bodies make up the *holosoma* (holo + soma), or set of bodies of the consciousness. The state of equilibrium or homeostasis of the holosoma directly influences the health of the consciousness.

4. **Multiexistentiality:** the consciousness has already had other previous lives and will be reborn again, with different genders, ethnic groups, and nationalities, drawing from human life the experiences and learning necessary for their evolution. Lives in the intraphysical dimension are interspersed by periods in the extraphysical dimension, called *intermissive periods*, in which the consciousness continues to act and manifest themselves, without the physical body. After being reborn, when the consciousness receives a new physical body, they are also called an *intraphysical consciousness (conscin)*. At the end of life, when the consciousness discards this body through biological death, they are called an *extraphysical consciousness (consciex)*.

5. **Intermissive Course:** during intermissive periods, consciousnesses can participate in *intermissive courses*, in order to qualify themselves for the best use of the next human life.

6. **Existential program:** human lives allow the consciousness to experience evolutionary experiences for themselves and others. When these experiences are planned in advance in a detailed and careful manner, the consciousness makes a commitment with themselves to perform the *existential program (proexis)*.

7. **Thosenity:** the basic manifestation of the consciousness is expressed with a thought or idea, which is always accompanied by a sentiment or emotion and a pattern of energy similar to this thought. This inseparable *thought-sentiment-energy* reality is called

a *thosene*. The set of *thosenes* characteristic of a consciousness, community, institution or environment, is called *holothosene*.

8. **Cosmoethics:** it is the cosmic, multidimensional ethics or moral code that is located beyond the still intraphysical social or human ethic. *Cosmoethics* act in the manner of cosmic laws, which govern the consciential evolution of the universe, and within the level of maturity already reached by the consciousness.

9. **Self-research:** it is performed by the person themselves, when carrying out research about themselves and on subjects that relate to them. Its purpose is to increase self-knowledge, self-awareness and to encourage intraconsciential renewals or *recyclings* (*recins*) sought by the person.

10. **Principle of Disbelief (PD):** the consciousness is guided not to believe in anything, not even in what is written in books or is said in conscientiology activities. The purpose is to build personal knowledge from *self-experimentation*, valuing personal experiences, with discernment and self-criticism, and employing all available research instruments. We invite readers to practice the Principle of Disbelief:

Do not believe in anything, not even the information provided in this book. Experiment, experience and perform self-research on health and care.

As a new science, conscientiology has developed and uses its own language, with specific terms, or **neologisms**, to define its ideas[68]. The objective is to ensure the accuracy of the concepts adopted and avoid confusion with similar but different ideas from other areas of knowledge. The neologisms used in this work are compiled in the glossary at the end of the book.

At the same time, conscientiology does not deny what is already known and explained by other sources of knowledge, nor does it intend to be new in all its propositions, using **knowledge** already accumulated by humanity so far, and what is in continuous production. An example of this compilation of knowledge is presented in the book Projectiology[67], whose bibliography refers to 1,907 consulted works, from 18 different languages, helping to explain the universality of psychic phenomena experienced by the consciousness at various times and by different groups throughout history.

The originality of conscientiology is thus not in its object of study, which is the consciousness and everything that relates to it, but in its scientific proposal of conscious **self-experimentation**, detached from mystification and dogmatism.

By bringing the consciential perspective closer to everyday life, we observe that most people still do not realize how they **interact** with the energies of different environments, objects, other people and animals, which is then fed back to their own energetic patterns, feelings and thoughts. Although many people already admit such influences, they still act instinctively, without observing the nuances of these interactions and the effects on themselves, on their personal health and on those close to them. Acting in a lucid way becomes even less frequent when we consider the extraphysical reality, and the interaction with consciousnesses present in these dimensions. However, the effects on one continue to occur, regardless of whether the person admits or is able to discriminate such conditions.

In summary, the **energies** are there, everywhere, under continuous, intentional or accidental influence, from the actions of each consciousness. This fact is still ignored by the majority of humanity, which does not apply their lucid will towards qualifying their personal energies and those energies around them, nor do they use them to help other consciousnesses. Changing this condition depends only on the person, and their intimate willingness to experience and develop the conscious mastery of energies, through various existing techniques of which we highlight the Basic Mobilization of Energies (BME).

The BME is a set of energetic maneuvers aimed at loosening the energosoma and obtaining holosomatic homeostasis. This is reached by achieving a state of balance in all the bodies of manifestation, and parapsychic development[67:584]. It consists of three key **energetic maneuvers**:

1. **Closed circulation:** through the conscious control of energetic movements by your personal will, the energies are drawn from the head to the feet and hands, and return to the head. The speed of the energetic movement is accelerated, preferably until the consciousness reaches the Vibrational State (VS) when the energies vibrate, and activate the whole energosoma. The size, intensity, speed and duration of the closed circulation of Consciential Energies (CEs) vary according to your will. Among the useful applications of this maneuver, we highlight installing the VS, a condition that predisposes lucid projection; promotes detoxification and energetic deassimilation; heals mini disturbances in health; provides energetic self-defense; and promotes the achievement and maintenance of balance and self-motivation. Such a practice vibratingly reorganizes the environment, bringing deep well-being and a positive disposition to the consciousness.

2. **Exteriorization of energies:** the conscious release or transfer of your personal energies is promoted through the will. This maneuver promotes assistance to others through the donation of energies and the energetic cleaning of environments.

3. **Absorption of energies:** the uptake or interiorization of healthy energies is performed in a lucid manner by your personal will. It is then important to verify the quality of energies from the sur-

rounding environment, in objects and from people before absorbing the energies. Benefits include the self-overcoming of energetic gaps, which can be noticed by your recovery from tiredness or fatigue.

The application of the consciential paradigm demarcates a new approach to the field of health called **consciential health.** According to the Encyclopedia of Conscientiology, *"consciential health is the natural condition, dynamic state of equilibrium or quality of the consciousness regarding their personal well-being, holosomatic homeostasis and the harmonious relationship with holothosenes, constituting a resource for self-evolution"*[69][Translation].

Also called holosomatic health, consciential health can be studied from different **perspectives** to help understand the variables that compose it, and the cause-and-effect relationships that it establishes. However, this differentiation is didactic, and does not reproduce practical observation, as multiple perspectives interact systemically, resulting in integral health that is expressed by the consciousness.

The subtlety of these **interactions** may go unnoticed, but their effects are concrete and cumulative, tending at some point to be perceived in the physical body. Thus, spiritual cures and diseases of a non-physical origin are experienced by the person. The health condition related to each one of the consciousness' vehicles of manifestation can be called[69]:

1. **Physical** health or somatic health, referring to the anatomical and physiological systems of the human body.

2. **Bioenergetic** health or energosomatic health, relating to the energetic balance of the energosoma.

3. **Emotional** health or psychosomatic health, relating to the emotions and affectivity linked to the psychosoma.

4. **Mental** health or mentalsomatic health, referring to the lucidity, rationality and logic expressed by the mentalsoma.

Another aspect relevant to consciential health is **parapsychic health**[69], which expresses the balance and well-being related to the *paraperceptions* of the consciousness, commonly known as extrasensory perceptions, regarding their multidimensional reality. *Parapsychism*, when applied lucidly, increases your self-knowledge and access to information regarding the conditions that influence your personal health and other consciousnesses, for example, through the following seven experiences:

1. The perception of **influences** from different environments and consciousnesses with which the person interacts, whether they are intraphysical or extraphysical, causing illnesses and remission.

2. The **inspiration** provided by more evolved consciousnesses regarding the care of your health, through *therapeutic insights* for yourself or others.

3. The conscious **absorption** of energies from more homeostatic environments.

4. The study of your personal health condition experienced in other **lives**, helping you to understand your current health in this life.

5. The research of your personal **temperament**, identifying the relationship between your evolutionary needs, growth crises and diseases.

6. The use of **lucid projection**, also known as astral projection or the conscious departure from the human body, in order to understand the non-physical perspective of your personal or other reality, thus better assisting your health.

7. The parapsychic experiences experienced by the person, which also allow them to know about their **immortal** reality, and

achieve the intimate certainty that after their death they will continue to exist, and have new physical lives, and new evolutionary opportunities. This fact frees the consciousness from the fear of death (thanatophobia), the root of all fears.

As already pointed out, the concept of consciential health is not intended to be totally new, because immaterial influences on health conditions have been addressed since antiquity through different areas of knowledge. The intention in this case is to assist consciousnesses to **construct** a multiexistential and multidimensional view, in order to boost their self-knowledge and self-research. Consequently, expanding their understanding of the meaning and interrelations in health, with scientificity and discernment.

Thus, by making holosomatic balance and the relationship with the different holothosenes in which each consciousness interacts **tangible**, consciential health makes the invisible relationships between health, the energies and thosenes that manifest or surround each consciousness objective.

Principles of Consciential Health

To understand consciential health, it is important to observe the principles that govern its action, in the form of universal laws, **foundations** or precepts. Just as physics postulates laws to explain the functioning of the universe, as exemplified by Newton's laws and the laws of thermodynamics, these principles seek to demonstrate how the health of the consciousness works.

However, such principles often contradict traditional logic, the biomedical model, personal beliefs and general culture. Knowing them is, therefore, inviting yourself to look at health from another **angle,** inserting new perspectives that alter your understanding, conclusions and attitudes regarding your experienced health condition. The following lists 11 principles of consciential health that support a greater understanding of the topic:

1. **Personal nature.** Consciential health is very personal, when expressing the consciential, complex and integral reality of the consciousness.

Health is not, then, an ancillary entity, external to the consciousness, but a facet of its **personality** and its experiences accumulated so far.

This perspective invites the person to **take charge** of their own health, as part of the whole, without separating or isolating health from the individual. It is inconsistent, in this view, to de-personify the disease by repelling it, excluding it from the self, or jettisoning it from the evolutionary process. Or even blaming the individual for their illness, for being who they are.

The effect is well expressed in the popular Chinese saying "there are no diseases, only sick people". Therefore, while it is important to group and categorize health and disease to advance in health research, it is not possible to reduce the individual to his or her disease, as both are integrated and extremely personal. There are no reliable **generalizations** in terms of human health[70].

Health and disease are not, therefore, *things* to be delegated to a health care professional, for their professional care, but **characteristics** of the individual themselves, to be managed by themselves with the support of health professionals. In this context, the individual is a specialist of themselves, and a generalist in health and disease conditions; while the professional is a specialist in health and disease conditions, and a generalist regarding the reality of the consciousness to be attended.

2. **Self-healing.** Consciential health is achieved through self-
-healing.

Strictly speaking, every **heterocure** is palliative and transitory, because it does not transform the intimate reality of the consciousness. Only when the consciousness faces the root causes of their consciential ailments, and recycles them, do they consolidate the intimate change that produces self-healing.

There are small self-healings, for example, when the person mobilizes their energies to install the vibrational state and dissipates the headache they felt, resulting from an assimilation of disharmonious energies; even larger self-healings, when the person intimately **modifies** the way they react to stress, reducing the irritability and tensions that triggered the headaches.

Self-healing is supported by **heterohelp**. However, sharing health decisions with a professional or family member is a choice to be made sparingly, since it is not possible to transfer personal responsibility for self-care to another person, no matter how great the reliance and competence may be. Thus, the more lucid the consciousness is, the more they choose, whenever possible, health professionals who support them in self-care actions, through reflective dialogue that promotes self-knowledge and personal recycling.

The **autonomy** regarding a person's personal decisions about their health, therefore, becomes an imperative, since only they will know how to reconcile the therapeutic options with their willingness to change, as well as meet their needs and objectives.

3. **Relativism.** Consciential health is relative, partial, imperfect, with a certain percentage of imbalance[71: 1507].

As far as we know, there is no final line or absolute health condition to be achieved. This characteristic represents the very evolution of the consciousness which, from a conscientiological perspective, does not have a known end, but **sequential stages**. At this point, we do not know the evolutionary process in its entirety, however, based on the principle that there is knowledge that is beyond human understanding, those themes constitute a mateology that will be understood in the future.

There is, therefore, no perfection in health, only continuous **improvement**. Health goals are outlined by the consciousness, to achieve the best relative health, considering their possibilities, needs and desires. The lucid planning of their health condition allows for *scheduled upgrades* that are tailored to their desired purposes.

Seeking perfection in health is, in itself, unhealthy[72]. The unbalanced pursuit of health can become an **obsession**, triggering mental disorders and severely restricting one's daily routine and social life. An obsession with healthy foods or orthorexia, for example, commonly triggers nutritional disorders due to the extreme selectivity of impure food options, and isolation when voluntarily excluding oneself from social activities involving food. Another less rare condition is the suffering generated by the disorder popularly known as a cleaning compulsion, in which the person spends a great deal of time meticulously cleaning, avoids going to places beyond the home, is at risk of getting skin sores and allergies due to the excessive use of products, and has a weakened personal immunity. And there is also the challenge of defining the limits between aesthetics and health, which imprison thousands of people in a cycle of consumption and frustration, in the search for unattainable standards of beauty and youth.

4. **Dynamism.** Consciential health is dynamic and, therefore, is in continuous transformation, following the context of life and changes in a consciousness.

It is a state of **equilibrium** that can be broken at any time, which does not necessarily mean an evolutionary delay or a setback in integral health. Illnesses and worsening health can paradoxically be evolutionary drivers in many cases.

The disease, often creates an opportunity for **reflection** on one's life and personal values. It recovers in the person the notion of finitude concerning this human existence and the search for meaning and purpose in their life. Acute or chronic illnesses can thus be the trigger for the adoption of healthier postures and intimate recycling, which favor execution of the proexis.

The emergence of difficulties and problems can also make the person realize the need to change for the better, and overcome aspects of themselves. These are moments of an **evolutionary** crisis, which may precipitate the appearance or exacerbation of diseases, just as they occur in the crises of the human life cycle, as represented by marriage, children and the empty nest syndrome[73].

Diseases act in this context, just like the *breaking of waves* in the sea, which needs to be overcome, to achieve a new phase of *calmness* or stabilization in one's life. However, **overcoming** it requires greater effort to face the inner resistance and turbulence of personal difficulties to achieve self-overcoming.

The search for the recovery of health thus increases self-perception, self-care and reinforces the value of human life for the person. Here, the disease acts as a **stabilizer** of personal health, contributing to balanced self-conviviality.

5. **Adaptability.** Consciential health is adaptable to the challenges and actions that the consciousness proposes to perform.

Since some **challenges** are stressors to their own health, the person temporarily renounces a part of their health to achieve a greater goal. The desired health outcome is not, in this case, the best possible one to be achieved, but is the one that balances the person's basic needs with their life purpose.

This situation occurs when the person does not allow themselves to stay in the **comfort zone** and sets goals in line with their existential program, which, nevertheless, provokes them to face their difficulties and partially abdicate their well-being to help others.

However, such lucid self-sacrifice does not mean self-flagellation or victimization. The **cosmoethical concession**, made by a consciousness, respects their fundamental needs, and is in harmony with their context of life. What reigns here is the *paralogic*, beyond human logic, which is capable of integrating the physical reality with the extraphysical one, and composing the multidimensional reality that directs the choices of the consciousness.

6. **Resource.** Consciential health is a pro-evolutionary resource, to be applied by a consciousness in multiple ways to optimize their evolution.

Health is therefore not an end in itself, but a resource whose good use and application depends on the **purpose** of one's personal life. And knowing one's life goals defines how much health a person will need to achieve them.

To embrace disease and its effects increases the consciousness' self-knowledge about their own completeness, constituting a resource to deepen **self-research** and boost their personal recycling and renewal. For this reason, "the best health comes after the illness and not before"[74:908][Translation]. Illness: self-assistantial opportunity.

There are diseases that force the person to stop, slow down their own life, to accept help, to renounce pleasures and running away, to review relationships, to adjust their direction in life, to change their environment, work or country, to review their choices, and in this way they invite **change**. Another person's illness can also be instigating, by requiring us to look at the people around us and granting our time, energy and resources to help them.

The existence of a disease thus causes each individual to move away from **automatism**, take a necessary stop for introspection and to redefine their priorities. They act as consciential symptoms, signaling intimate needs that are begging to be met.

Unlike the religious-based western view that historically associates disease with punishment, the disease becomes a tool and, in some cases, even a **gift** or opportunity.

This is the case of the **disease** that arises during a deviation of the proexis, allowing for an adjustment to the life path; one that demands a dedicated routine, which stabilizes the daily life of the person[75:390]; that brings people back together who have broken relationships, and promotes reconciliation; that reactivates inner conflicts, fostering recycling and the attainment of a higher evolutionary level; and the one that produces the catharsis of conflicts accumulated by the consciousness in this and other lives, providing the release of stagnant and blocked energies.

Often, a fatalistic and negative **perspective** of diseases causes more suffering than the actual limitation and symptoms of the disease itself. By reviewing its meaning, and building a more positive view of the disease, the person has more energy to invest in their own self-healing. Self-victimizing or blaming others for the loss of your health is wasted time.

Alternatively, we cannot sanctify diseases, since there are always **risks** and potential deleterious effects to life. Therefore, it is reasonable to consider that some diseases are manifested under the technical assistance of *extraphysical helpers*, extraphysical consciousnesses specialized in multidimensional assistance, who technically help the person concerned to contain the harmful effects on their health, especially when such diseases promote important positive effects for the person and the group around them.

7. **Syncretism.** Consciential health is syncretic and transdisciplinary, using multiple areas of knowledge without restricting itself to the divisions of knowledge categorized by humanity.

By critically analyzing the contributions from many different areas of health, and the knowledge produced so far, the best of each approach is sought and **gathered** together, without ruling any of them out based on a priori reasoning.

The multiplicity of health practices, structured from several paradigms, expands the therapeutic options that can be experienced by the professional and the patient. Different therapies can bring equivalent gains to an individual's personal health, because there is more than one **way** to solve a problem. And, when therapies become associated with one another, they can produce complementary and synergistic effects that restore the condition of personal balance.

8. **Integrality.** Consciential health is integral, and composes all facets of a consciousness in all dimensions in which they manifest.

A person's own health does not end with **death**, because it accompanies the consciousness who continues to manifest themselves in intermissive periods. It is carried from one life to another and thus each consciousness brings their previous experiences with them, including their *para*sicknesses, *para*scars, *para*diseases and *para*syndromes.

Thus, health is not restricted to the **soma**, but extrapolates its condition, and paradoxically there may be weak physical health associated with relatively balanced consciential health. This occurs close to death, for example, when the body is already weakened, but the consciousness is elated at having completed the challenges of their proexis that they undertook to perform, or even, in some cases, have accomplished beyond what was proposed.

Another paradoxical case is the self-programmed disease, which happens when the consciousness lucidly plans, before birth, to have a disease that amplifies their interassistantial potential. In this context, the disease becomes a **facilitator**, rather than an obstacle to the desired goals. An extreme example of this condition studied in conscientiology is the *Serenissimus* Reurbanizer, who was born oligophrenic, it seems, to be able to devote himself to multidimensional assistance practically full time, while outsourcing his care to other people and sparing him from traditional social routines[74:374].

Even if such examples seem distant, this principle applies to the personal context, reinforcing the idea that no single aspect of health can be considered a global **measure** of the consciousness. The relativization of what we conventionally associate with *being healthy* encourages us to broaden our understanding about health.

The health of the soma, as opposed to being the predominant element, is the most **rustic**, dense and palpable expression of the integral health of the consciousness. Taking care of our own soma, however difficult, is just *the start of the beginning* of the journey. Somatic imbalances can be compensated or even cured by consciential health[1:1346] because, ultimately, the health of the soma is maintained from the holosoma's homeostasis.

9. **Prophylaxis.** Consciential health is prophylactic, preventive, and acts in accordance to the popular expression that "prevention is better than the cure".

Prophylaxis begins with the **thosene**, from the *tho* element, thoughts produced by the consciousness, are charged with sentiments and energies of an equivalent pattern, and are magnetized in all the bodies or vehicles of manifestation. Cosmoethical thinking, with logic and linear intentions, called an *orthothosene*, is the greatest pharmacy of the consciousness.

Prophylaxis is nourished by healthy **habits** and useful routines, that maintain the consciousness' minimum threshold of relative health, despite the overloads and excesses present in everyday life.

It also works as a personal health savings account, in which the goods of health are accumulated, managed and drawn with lucidity by the consciousness, who decides when it is time to **invest** their personal health into some evolutionary project. The consciousness evaluates the risks and potential benefits for themselves and everyone else, defining the appropriate moment to give up part of their already earned relative health for an action that will generate *evolutionary dividends* and garner greater consciential health in the future. Such contemplation measures the minimum level of health the consciousness needs to maintain for the survival of their soma and the balance of their other vehicles.

10. **Exemplarism.** Consciential health is exemplary, and it positively inspires the people around us, in the interest of reaching a similar level of harmony and intimate tranquility.

Our **own example** reverberes and transforms people, from a spontaneous social dynamic, and constitutes a powerful means of mutual assistance or *inter*assistance. An aura of health emitted by the consciousness is intuitively perceived by the other people around them, awakening sensations in all vehicles of manifestation, with physical, energetic, emotional and mental repercussions. The effects can vary from irresistible attraction and wanting to come closer to this consciousness to uncontrollable repulsion, qualifying the degree of affinity and interest among consciousnesses.

There is also the case of consciousnesses with a lower level of health that, when achieving something that is evolutionarily beneficial, **provoke** other consciousnesses to review their own evolutionary efforts, acting as a *pebble in a shoe*, urging those in good health to redouble their efforts.

The expression of **health** in each body, with exemplary effects, can be synthesized by the trivocabular megathosenes proposed by Vieira[1:624]: "*Self-disposition: somatic health. Self-megaeuphorization: energosomatic health. Megafraternity: psychosomatic health. Self-discernment: mentalsomatic health. Serenology: holosomatic health*" [Translation].

11. **Assistantiality.** Consciential health is assistantial, altruistic, and built from helping other consciousnesses. In the area of health, "the best remedy that exists is to help others."[m]

The **purpose** of interassistance mobilizes the person to help others, to increase their perception of themselves and others, and to enable them to provide care. It accelerates the individual's own evolution, encouraging them to learn from the experiences of other consciousnesses.

By allowing themselves to become immersed in the difficulties faced by other consciousnesses, the person reviews the size of their problems, dedramatizes their consciential reality and places the focus of their attention away from themselves to help those who have a greater problem than their own. This means giving up the position of victim to be a protagonist of their own and the group's health at all levels. Assistance thus becomes an **input** to cure all evils.

---

m Speech of Dr. Waldo Vieira during the tertulia about behavioral systematization, on February 22, 2010, available at: https://www.youtube.com/watch?v=1eaWJ1tavPc

The continued practice of assisting others expands the **technicality** of the consciousness' assistance, preparing them to act in the role of *extraphysical helper*, both in the physical and extraphysical dimensions, to conscins and consciexes.

Have you *considered* some of the *principles* of consciential health to better **understand** your ***health-disease process***? *Do you apply your energies,* in a **conscious** way, for the benefit of your health? Have you already used your **parapsychism** to *help improve your health and that of others*?

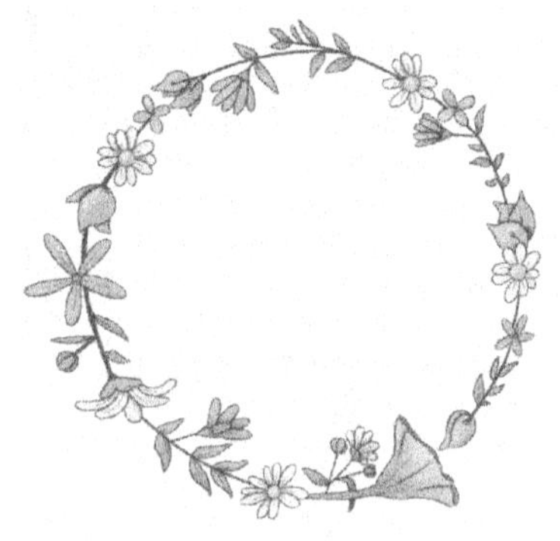

Chapter 4
Research in Health

"Science is not a formal construction, but an activity
realized by research communities."
Ludwik Fleck (1896–1961)

How is health research carried out? How do you *research* or search for *evidence* in health? How do the *results* of this research *change the care and assistance* you offer and receive? The objectives of this chapter are to address how **health knowledge** is produced, in different paradigms, and to critically analyze the **impacts** of this research on **health care**, both for professionals and patients.

At the beginning of this book, we spoke about the evolution of health and care conceptions by addressing different health paradigms. In this chapter, our focus will be on health **research**, because it is closely linked to what is recognized as being healthy and doing what is healthy. Research also interacts with the health practices and resources offered, based on trends and fads.

Health care has become a large market in which the scientific support for products is given weight from the results of the studies carried out. However, scientific research is interspersed with **limitations**, biases and interests. Understanding this context favors both professionals and individuals in general in the interpretation and practical application of the published health results.

To begin with, let's resume the discussion on paradigms and health sciences based on **Cartesian thinking** and the search for truth through reason. In the Book Discourse on Method, the French philosopher and mathematician René Descartes presented the possibility of obtaining indubitable knowledge that could be reproduced collectively, without being dogmatic, but rather in a free and methodical manner. Thus, he demonstrated that there is an experience that leads to the truth in the method and defended this way of making science as a liberating activity, capable of freeing society from truths considered dogmatic or eternal[76].

In this direction, the Modern Era walked, recognizing method and reason as a dominant scientific rationality. **Science** can thus be understood as the "set of methodically acquired knowledge, more or less systematically organized, and capable of being transmitted by a pedagogical teaching process"[77:43][Translation].

Scientific advances influenced the production of knowledge and the development of technological innovations. In the early 1950's, however, scientific knowledge was established with a **preference for the process** in relation to the research content[78]. At the end of the 20th century, this condition influenced a dependence on science for technological development, which was not accompanied by reflection on the ethical repercussions of this process[79].

Scientificity, in addition to rigid models and standards, should be thought of as a highly abstracted regulatory idea that relates theory and empirical reality, by means of method[80]. From this perspective, science is conceived as a method to guide the study and practice of disciplines, which varies in cyclical time periods and should not be considered as an unquestionable value. It must therefore be constantly debated, especially regarding the difficulty of observing the human as an inseparable being. Its primary objective is thus to produce knowledge and circulate it in networks[81].

In this sense, the philosophy researcher Chris **Lawn**[82] argues that if the fixation of science remains in the method, alternative forms of seeking truth may be overshadowed, in addition to influencing in the sphere of human sciences a restrictive vision of man as a purely rational (and material) being. After all, objective reason tends to subordinate people to a single way of seeing the world[83].

If, on the one hand, the appropriation of reason into the scientific method developed science by making it overcome unverifiable **truths**, on the other hand, it has restricted the ability to understand man as an inherently subjective being. Recovering this subjectivity demands a broader perspective of science, as a producer of knowledge about the objective-subjective and tangible-intangible *continuum* that integrates humans.

Gadamer, like other philosophers of the 20th century, also criticized scientific rationalism, since one cannot think of truth only in relation to reason[82]. Gadamer proposed the experience of dialogue through the use and appropriation of language, as a way to find the truth. One can seek to trace through language how people understand the world or their state of health. For Gadamer, the communicative dimension of language is one of the most powerful means of putting a human being in contact with another, leading them to recognize themselves each and every time[84].

Making **language** circular allows for greater emancipation of the person, and can thus make society rethink its role in the world. However, no method or concept guarantees the truth, if understood as a form of relationship with oneself and between people. Therefore, looking for mechanisms that favor the use of language in genuine dialogue can be a process of seeking the truth[83,84].

We are born into a world full of meaning in which language does not always seek the truth because it is dependent on **humans**[84]. The search for the truth will depend on overcoming human weaknesses and systematic distortions of communication concerning certain interests, based on intentionality, temperament and personal traits. Thus, the importance of rational dialogue in the practice and production of knowledge is recovered.

The German philosopher and sociologist **Habermas**[85,86] also proposes language as an instrument for understanding the world based on the experience of phenomena, as a way of going beyond cognitive-instrumental rationality, and achieving communicative rationality. For the author:

> "the phenomenon to be explained is not the knowledge or submission of an objectified nature taken by itself, but the intersubjectivity of the possible understanding, both on the interpersonal plane and on the intrapsychic plane"[85:499,500][Translation].

The model of science constitutes the dominant explanation scheme in industrialized societies, considered more plausible and intellectually accepted, however it is by no means exclusive[87]. Since science has failed to produce sufficient truths for a fast-paced world that continually lacks answers, and since there are no absolute truths, **gaps** have been created to resolve problems, as such creating crises in the contemporary world in relation to the production of knowledge.

An exclusively **quantitative** production of knowledge limits one's ability to grasp the nature of the patient's world and care. The alternative is to prepare professionals to build knowledge from different methodological approaches that bring them closer to their research object, the patient. And in this way, it enables clinical practice to advance[88].

To this end, Turato[89] proposes the consideration of research methods that use resources other than numbers, percentage calculations, statistical techniques, tables, numerically representative samples, random trials, closed questionnaires or evaluation scales; characteristic of the quantitative method. In the **qualitative** methodology applied to health, the conception brought from the human sciences should be used, according to which

> "the aim is not to study the phenomenon itself, but to understand its individual or collective meaning in people's lives. It is therefore essential to know what the phenomena of illness and life in general represent for them. *Meaning* has a structuring function: in terms of what things mean, people will somehow organize their lives, including their own health care" [89:509][Translation].

Understanding the meaning of **phenomena** regarding the health-disease process is essential to[89]:

1. Improve the quality of the professional-patient-family-institution **relationship**.

2. Promote greater **adherence** of patients and the population to individually administered treatments and collectively implemented measures.

3. Understand more deeply certain feelings, ideas and **behaviors** of patients, as well as their relatives and even the professional health team.

The evolution of **qualitative** research allows one to expand the format of the research. However, the quantitative-qualitative dichotomy remains without an outcome, especially in relation to the validity, rigor and reliability of qualitative research. Nonetheless, in addition to seeking new evaluation criteria, each study can also be considered as unique and individual, and can be evaluated on its own merits[90,91].

An alternative to approaching quantitative and qualitative methods in a systematized way is the **mixed methods** research. This method values the differences in paradigms between the methods, as long as their delimitations and differences are clear, thus enabling a rigorous conversation between fields[92].

This approach is fundamental, because neither of the two approaches is more scientific than the other. Scientific knowledge is always a link between a theory and an empirical reality, and the method is the common thread to form this connection. In this context, the limitation of **evidence-based** medicine should be understood. In the current model of science production, favoring quantitative findings as an authority to guide decision-making in health, without valuing the results of qualitative studies, can be a barrier to understanding health problems.

It is understood, however, that there are strategic moments when the quantitative knowledge obtained from the study of the cause-effect relationship should be applied, for example, in the control of **epidemics** or in the urgency and emergency approach. But this use is not enough for all areas of health, since it is not possible to restrict the world of life by the prevailing Cartesian and dominant systemic rationale[83,84].

In bringing the **qualitative** research debate to the health field, researcher Maria Cecília Minayo[87] points out that the expansion of theoretical and methodological conceptual bases does not make the health sciences less scientific, but, to the contrary, it brings them closer to the phenomena studied and to the production of knowledge.

In this sense, **language** is essential to understand the phenomena and to recover a reflective practice, without idealizations or norms, since there is no ideal care, but rather an exchange of knowledge among those involved in the process and who together will be able to make the best decisions. Language will be more valid the more it encourages dialogue, as a way of relating to a particular subject, with oneself and with others.

The **proposal** is not to do away with reason, but to recover a broader understanding of the life sciences by uniting theory and practice to improve the worldview, relationships and experiences of the people involved.

Therefore, for health practices in general, we propose for the person to seek the dialogical construction of reason in their investigative practice that is less mechanistic-normative and more focused on care, while valuing experiences that allow for understanding the complexity of the human being. Thus, scientific evolution can be facilitated in all segments of the study. And, in the case of health, this **maturation** is implemented through changes in thinking and care practice, influencing the quality of care provided to patients. However, these changes, even though they represent advances in care, have not always been or are easily incorporated by health professionals and patients.

If we look back at history, it took more than 100 years for discoveries on how to prevent **scurvy** at sea to be implemented as a health protection measure. In 1601, English captain James Lancaster discovered that adding three spoons of lemon juice to the sailors' diet completely reduced their chance of getting sick from the disease. However, it was only in 1795 that the English Navy adopted this practice for its vessels[93].

It can be seen, therefore, that there are several influencing factors for **knowledge** to be incorporated into health practices. In the case of vitamin C, just discovering the benefits of its use was not enough for the rapid diffusion and application of this knowledge. In addition, new researchers and experiences were needed to eliminate scurvy from the merchant navy[93].

Until 1900, it took humanity about 100 years to double its accumulated knowledge. In the middle of the 20th century, this time decreased to 25 years. Today, this knowledge doubles every 18 months. Although there is no consensus among the **metrics** used to measure this growth, whose variables include subject areas, time periods, types of publication and locations, the increase in research is remarkable[94].

Access to research has also been expanded in recent decades, especially by computerization. However, it is difficult for the healthcare professional to keep up to date, with so much research and so many **publications**. In the area of integrative and complementary practices, for example, there are currently more than 1 million scientific studies in the Virtual Health Library on Traditional, Complementary and Integrative Medicines (VHL TCIM)[n]. The large number of studies creates a challenge for any researcher in this field.

To facilitate access to available evidence and identify gaps in knowledge, review methods were developed to synthesize the knowledge produced. Health **reviews** provide the best clinical decision-making, favoring the planning and administration of health

n   http://mtci.bvsalud.org/en/

services, the definition of policies and programs to be implemented, and the definition of new research strategies[95].

There are 14 more common types of reviews, in which the **evidence map** method stands out, as it uses graphical (or dynamic, via interactive *online* databases) representations that facilitate the interpretation of results[96]. Returning to the example of complementary therapies, clinical evidence maps about them[o] present research that is available in the VHL and other databases. Thus, evidence maps become useful tools for decision-making for managers, health professionals and patients[97].

In this dynamic scenario, it is estimated that the current average time to implement a scientific discovery for the benefit of society is 17 years[98]. However, the **distance** between research and practice goes beyond the temporal question, because safety and effectiveness issues continue to be challenges for the translation of knowledge, especially when the evidence is not demonstrated through quantitative studies, as is the case of many health practices that also took more than a century to be recognized.

In 1854, **Florence Nightingale**, who is considered the first theorist in the field of nursing, recommended the use of lavender essential oil (*Lavandula angustifolia)* on the forehead of soldiers wounded during the Crimean War to calm them down. But it was only in 1997 that the Brazilian Federal Nursing Council included some alternative practices as a specialty. And in 2016, Gnatta and collaborators[99] recovered this part of history and connected this practice with nursing theories, contributing to the dissemination and implementation of aromatherapy as a healthcare practice in the profession. Implicitly, it also retrieved Florence's ideas that consid-

---

o   https://mtci.bvsalud.org/en/evidence-map/

ered nursing as an art, a healing process, which should put the patient in the best condition for nature to act on them.

Thus, the concept of health proposed by the great Greek philosophers, such as Aristotle, Plato and Hippocrates, is recovered: health is understood not as something that the physician brings by themselves, but as something that can only happen through the physician helping **nature** to cure itself[100].

Health in this sense is understood as a state of **balance** and the role of the health team is understood as a facilitator of the care process, which is not restricted to symptom control. According to Ayres[84], the caring attitude must expand to all reflections and interventions in the field of health.

To achieve this condition, we must seek to change how the production of knowledge is developed by linking truth with language, as well as seek to understand health from the **meaning** people attribute to this phenomenon. Moreover, from a multidimensional perspective, this involves abandoning the idea of disease as just a morphofunctional disorder, with a view to individualizing care, and understanding the dynamic balance as having the potential to improve our health and life.

Based on this understanding, it is necessary to include reason, language and phenomenon in the conception of a paradigm, as a model to be relativized, allowing us to understand the process of change from a systematic and complex perspective. This perspective should guide health research in the search for truth, based on different quantitative, **qualitative and mixed** research designs, and will also benefit from research on integrative and complementary practices and on consciential health, which contribute to rethinking our health paradigms.

Research in Integrative Health

Health research provokes constants **clashes** between health professionals and complementary therapies, because it is complex to research, within the parameters of biomedical science, different medical rationales and practices based on other paradigms. Many times, the methodologies accepted by the scientific community, especially the western one, are not adequate tools for evaluating these therapies.

As a result, potential barriers to conduct research in complementary therapies are identified, such as the different concepts of health and disease, a lack of agreement between diagnostic criteria, contrasting views on the therapeutic process and **different theories** about the etiology of diseases.

The mere transference of the conception of Western scientific research, according to positivist principles, may be at odds with the holistic foundations on which complementary therapies are structured. There would be many more problems in terms of the paradigm, a transition from different worldviews, and the challenge of **integrating** this knowledge, than the actual lack of evidence and clinical effectiveness of these practices[101].

One of the difficulties is to perform clinical studies that consider **individualization** and subjective factors present in complementary therapies. Bioscience and its harder parts have been recognized as the only one to produce truths about health and disease, monopolizing the training of specialists and being fed back by a fragmented form of research[102], such as studying only one physiological response or one health outcome.

In studies on **homeopathy**, for example, even if the results are favorable, they were not enough to change the scientific community regarding the difficulty of framing homeopathic knowledge and practice within the biomedical theoretical body[102].

In **phytotherapy,** the most numerous and growing studies have an ethnobotanic and pharmacological focus and objective. However, these studies bring the risk that the use of plants in more fragile non-industrialized forms will be progressively replaced by synthetic drugs and industrialized herbal medicine. This replacement would discourage the dissemination of relatively safe and simple knowledge of the popular and professional use of native plants, *in natura* or with local handmade manipulation, to Primary Health Care professionals and the population[102].

One way to conduct research in complementary therapies is to seek its institutional legitimization through science, using quantitative methodologies and laboratory studies. Another way to contest scientific dogmatism is to build "social wisdom" in order to **value** what is not currently recognized as science and, through political, social and institutional action, break its influence over what it identifies as important or not. And, in this way, truths and efficiencies can be recognized in ways that are different from Western medicine, based on their own criteria, "through a scientific approach that seeks detachment and the relativization of official medicine"[102:271][Translation].

The analysis of experiences from complementary therapies and the development of methodology approaches with the institutional universe of complementary therapies, "a kind of research action or evaluation of a participatory nature, can contribute to greater **visibility** and an institutional breakdown of research, in addition to the production of knowledge and its academic circulation"[102:278][Translation].

Therefore, to carry on research in complementary therapies requires considering the different classification criteria for diseases, its causes and its evolution, which are often highly **artisanal** and individualizing in terms of diagnosis and treatment, and thus divergent from Western medicine[102].

Different **methodologies** and study designs seek to bring researchers closer to the reality experienced by people and communities, and to produce knowledge that truly meets the needs of patients, health professionals and managers. Comparative effectiveness surveys[103] are examples of these methodologies that seek to compare the benefits and harm of alternative methods, including from new drugs to complementary therapies, to prevent, diagnose, treat and monitor a clinical condition or to improve the provision of care, focusing on the relationship between health professionals and patients.

Clinical trials are valuable safety and **efficacy** regulators, but they are also voice silencers of patients and healthcare professionals. Relations of trust, the senses, words, gestures, relationships and care in contact with the healing professional need to be valued more in health research[102].

Part of the treatment in complementary therapies is related to the individualization of care and development of the patient's **empowerment** over their state of health and illness. Therefore, to think of the placebo effect as a result of the professional-patient relationship (or in the case of research, researcher-object of the study) is to consider that this moment of exchange in the medical office (research space) is relevant to the care process.

Many changes have occurred in the process of producing knowledge related to complementary therapies. For example, 50 years ago, **meditation** was considered quackery, and the possibility of it being considered a medical treatment sounded absurd. However, the development of scientific studies and the mapping of physiological changes brought about by these practices have changed this scenario. Currently, mind-body therapies, a type of complementary therapy that combines mental focus, controlled breathing and body movements, are growing in popularity[104].

Historically, these practices have been used to promote flourishing, awareness, peace, enlightenment, and human connection. Today, many people are attracted to these practices for their perceived physical and mental **benefits** in health and stress relief[104]. Thus, it is questioned which factors were instrumental in generating this paradigm shift.

However, there are still difficulties in recognizing the **preventive** potential of mind-body medicine, due to the limitation of seeing this care process within a treatment model that is predominantly built with a focus on disease reaction[104]. Therefore, it is essential to explore how changes in the process of producing health knowledge occur, which favor the expansion of the preventive application of these practices.

Science from the Fleck Perspective

The process and production of knowledge has been widely studied by Polish physician-philosopher Ludwik **Fleck**. His vision is in tension with the positivist model, in which research is isolated from the researcher, and in which truth exists for itself, thus helping us to understand the intrinsic relationship between the knowledge produced and the community that produces it. His pioneering work has influenced researchers, historians, sociologists and philosophers of science, such as Thomas Kuhn, and is still thought provoking today. To understand his ideas, it is important that we familiarize ourselves with the concepts he proposes, some of which are considered precursors and similar to Michel Foucault's notions of épistémè, and Thomas Kuhn's paradigm[105].

For Fleck, **knowledge** is a social activity par excellence and cannot be understood as an individual act[106]. It is thought by a group of people and composes their Thought Style (TS), which is defined as the way of seeing, understanding and conceiving from a certain bio-psycho-social context[107]. Each set of people are called a Thought Collective (TC), and they are characterized as a community of people that gathers and conditions the knowledge of a given TS. The TC are established through esoteric circles, formed by groups of scientists who produce knowledge, while interacting with exoteric circles, being the source community for production and a consumer of the knowledge produced.

In Fleck's view, a well-organized **collective** is a bearer of knowledge that far surpasses the capacity of any individual, since the social structure favors an organized effort in the division of tasks, collaboration and the reciprocal exchange of ideas, among other advantages[108]. In effect, the TS almost always imposes a compulsory force on the thoughts of the individual bound to a collective, since they are rarely or almost never aware of the prevalent TS. The TS thus consists of a directed perception, predisposing the individual and the group to a selective feeling and to the consequent directed action.

Fleck is dedicated to demonstrating the importance of the density of interactions that occur in modern science, and which contribute to the stability and universality of Western science. Such interactions allow for the homogenization of ideas and practices and the creation of a ***harmony of illusions*** that first tries to adapt new knowledge to the scientific fact already accepted by the collective, or such knowledge will be effectively neutralized by this collective[109]. The neoconcepts proposed by Fleck are summarized in the following table:

Table 1. Description of the concepts proposed by Ludwik Fleck[106].

Concept	Description
Thought Collective	Science is something cooperatively accomplished and can be characterized by different groups and their Thought Styles.
Thought Style	A way of seeing, understanding and conceiving a body of knowledge and practices from a bio-psy-cho-socio-cultural context.
Change in Thought Style	It is the fundamental process for the progress of knowledge to occur, being divided into three stages: 1) establishment of the new Thought Style; 2) extension — formation of concepts; 3) transformation — construction of the scientific fact.
Scientific fact	Historical-evolutionary theory of knowledge.
Esoteric circle	Producers of knowledge in relation to another Collective.
Exoteric circle	Source for the production of knowledge and consumers of the product in relation to another Thought Collective.
Coercion of thought	A way to regulate a Thought Style.
Historicity of knowledge	It admits a model of production of interactionist knowledge between subject and object and highlights the dialectical conception of truth.
Interdisciplinarity	Different Thought Collectives and Styles can interact in border zones — transitional spaces — for the construction of knowledge.
Harmony of illusions	Adaptation of new knowledge to those previously established, aiming to maintain a Thought Style.
Nuances	The intermediate view of the collective when the coexistence of different Thought Styles occurs.

Source: Löwy[109], Cutolo[107], Fleck[108].

For Fleck[108], **knowledge** is conceived as the human capacity to collectively discuss and analyze the relationships of human beings, themselves and the environment in which they live, in theory and in practice, and the result of the human social process since the beginning of civilization.

Fleck's ambitious goal was to develop a comparative **episte-mology**, such as a "science of science" that could explain how modern and contemporary sciences work, that is, describe how they are formed and relate to each other, and how this relationship cannot be separated from the culture and society in which they are inserted[109].

In this sense, scientific production that originates from research is fundamental for **maintaining** a Thought Style, since it allows for the circulation of knowledge between the esoteric and exoteric circles, and the coercion of thought.

According to Fleck[108], every scientific theory has a period of classicism, in which there are situations that fit perfectly into it, and another period of complications, where exceptions begin to appear, and, in the end, the persistence of the exceptions surpass the regular cases. At this moment, there is a **disruption of *the harmony of illusions*** and a new style becomes established in the Thought Collective. Thus, scientific renewal demands the accumulation of disastrous or exceptional results, which disqualify the established truth, and allow a new truth to emerge that can explain the new results found.

As an example of knowledge that promoted change in the Thought Styles of the collectives during its time, we can cite Charles **Darwin's** The Origin of Species, which first generated refutation and brought discredit to the author and later, had its proposed scientific fact validated and its due importance to science recognized.

The rupture of the *harmony of illusions*, as characterized by Fleck, does not occur in a linear manner among the researchers of a collective, but in an asymmetrical way, generating dissent and potential dissent. Updated for the current times, regarding the rapid propagation of knowledge in the information age, provides space for these **dissenters** to speak directly to exoteric circles of consumers through mass communication. This phenomenon has generated more and more heterogeneous knowledge and demanded greater criticism from people.

By applying **Fleck's theory** to the production of health knowledge, the different medical rationales and health practices comprise Thought Styles, formed by collectives that study and use these practices.

From this perspective, the knowledge produced and applied in Western medicine is as subjective, imprecise and participatory as that of other medical rationales and complementary therapies, because it represents the TS of the collective that builds and conditions it. These limitations of the scientific method in Western medicine are not only perceived when we are immersed in this TC, living in **harmony** with the *harmony of illusions*.

In this sense, for the progress of knowledge to occur, it is essential to foster **changes** in Thought Styles, based on a critical approach to what constitutes scientific knowledge. The legitimation of other TS's, through complementary therapies, is an alternative to broaden the perception of limitations and potentialities of each TS, inviting the different TC's to interact in border zones — transition spaces — for the construction of knowledge in an interdisciplinary way.

By the end of the 19th century, science had been divided into many disciplines and the search for interaction and the promotion of dialogue aroused an interest in **interdisciplinarity**, seeking deeper connections between the different fields of science. This movement could lead to transdisciplinarity, understood as a global integration of the sciences[110].

However, it is important to identify the degree of **autonomy** of each discipline during the integration and interaction between the different areas of knowledge. A positivist trap in the process is to try to analyze and understand the different areas of science from the same method or by using the same logic. As an example of this trap, Pereira[110] presents "the notorious and sometimes ideological appropriation of Darwin's concept of evolution over nature, which is applied to think about and understand society" [Translation].

In the 1950's, preventive medicine was freed from the notion of a single cause of disease, based on bacteriology, as it became unsustainable to explain disease as the effect of a pathogenic agent action only and, in turn, started to adopt the **multiple cause** model. From this moment onwards, the idea of a health team appeared to be supported mainly by the notion of integrative health care to the patient, however with a central role in the physician's work[111].

The expansion of community medicine required a new structuring of the elements that constituted medical practice, so as to incorporate complementary and interdependent work among the different health workers. Thus, **teamwork** is a response to the need for the integration of disciplines and professions, which is essential for the development of health practices based on the new biopsychosocial conception of the health-disease process[111].

Health practice can benefit from the **coexistence** of different styles and collectives, which embrace the varied worldviews, and seek to expand the health-disease-care process, especially if in this process they help to break the *harmony of illusions* of refractory and inhumane Thought Styles.

Science already has health research designs and tools that can help to modify the current biomedical paradigm, however, to expand this paradigm is to act in the counterflow and, more than evidence, it requires a **change in the posture** of researchers and health professionals, to:

1. Critically reflect on health and care concepts, in addition to the normative-ideal, supported by quantitative and qualitative research and various medical rationales and integrative and complementary practices.

2. Reconsider professional roles and the way of working, including an analysis of the financial interests in the health area, the use of cumulative, invasive and costly technologies for patients and health systems, the increasing medicalization of life, the limits of the current model to promote the empowerment of patients and the lack of therapeutic exemplarism.

3. Experience other health paradigms, whether from personal experiences or from the construction of care with patients, considering transcendental references to Western medicine, such as bioenergies, multidimensionality, the existence of various lives and the relationships between consciousnesses before this physical life.

To promote such changes in attitude, it is essential for professionals to get to know and experience the research process beyond the professional practice of health, and also to experience it in researching themselves, aiming to increase their understanding of the reality of other consciousnesses, and their own self-awareness, with a focus on **interassistance**.

Is the **research** that you use as a reference to *guide your health care* and practice *mostly quantitative, qualitative, or mixed*? Can you **identify** *the Thought Collectives and Thought Styles* that **converse** with your *health care and practice*?

Chapter 5
Relations between Health and Consciousness

> "There are times in life when the question of knowing if
> one can think differently than one thinks, and perceive
> differently than one sees, is absolutely necessary if one is to
> go on looking and reflecting at all."
> Michel Foucault (1926–1984)

To what extent is *health* an *expression of personal traits, temperament and your consciential essence*? How much can **health research** benefit from studying these relationships? The objectives of this chapter are to explain the *inseparable connections between health and the consciousness* and to present notions of **consciousness research** and the bases of *conscientiological research*.

We experience a great **paradox**: if, on the one hand, we want safe answers, which bring us certainties, in various fields of life, including health; on the other, we want individuality, and the freedom to think, experience and live with autonomy. But how can we build certainties in the midst of so much subjectivity? How can we replicate, standardize or obtain representation in scientific findings regarding such personal traits? Are we able to renounce the solidity of certainties and assume the fluidity of subjectivities inherent to our essence?

The relationship between health and the consciousness has been covered in this book, and here we are going to deepen our ability to critique the way knowledge is constructed about the consciousness that communicates with health research. An understanding of health involves understanding the human condition, in all its complexity, trends, virtues, setbacks, approaches, individuality and heterogeneity. But treading the path of investigating the consciousness requires appropriating the **intangible reality** that exists inside and outside of us.

The consciousness discussed in this chapter can have different **meanings**, depending on the paradigm used. It is the essence, being, ego, soul, self, personality, mind, psyche, among other synonyms. What is relevant is the trait of uncertainty, subjectivity and individuality that passes through all these meanings.

Social scientist Brené Brown[p] became known worldwide for researching the power of **vulnerability** and reframing the importance of other uncomfortable feelings, such as shame and fear, in the construction of socially valued characteristics such as courage, empathy, and leadership. Her current motto has been "courage above comfort", which invites change.

Conquering this positive and benevolent outlook in the face of personal frailties, in a crescendo that starts with curiosity, moves to interest and then reaches the genuine joy of being in front of something new and unknown, is feasible to any person. Here is the

---

p The author's presentation of the power of vulnerability is available at: https://www.ted.com/talks/brene_brown_the_power_of_vulnerability

opportunity to discover, experience and accomplish something that was once invisible. But this posture demands the **deconstruction** of models, beliefs, and values that are socially constructed and introjected in our minds. Some of which have been endorsed by authorities of science, morality or faith.

Reviewing **reference models** is essential for each one of us to rebuild our relationship with ourselves and, our health, to the extent that we are able to apply this same interest to the unknown in relation to our personal health. The worldview that permeates the relationship of the person with their health establishes the relationship with themselves as an expression of their consciousness.

Many traditional medicines that make up complementary therapies are also structured around this understanding that the body's functioning is continuously affected by the attitudes, sentiments and thoughts of the human being. Examples of this can be found in traditional Chinese medicine, anthroposophical medicine and Ayurvedic medicine. These varying medical perspectives promote an **expanded view** of being in the world *versus* a dual explanation common to current medicine, which divides actions and attitudes into right-wrong, good-evil, those that blame and those that seek to control the body.

Still, researchers who study the consciousness may ignore a relationship between health and the **consciousness**. As a result, this relationship will not be considered in their research and it will not be presented to professionals and patients who use the knowledge produced, thus restricting the benefits of a practice such as meditation to reduce stress, even though its subjective effects may include a better relationship with themselves and with life's uncertainties.

Building the foundation for **better health** that achieves benefits yet to be enjoyed, and integrates the personal characteristics of individuals, requires bringing together the concepts of health and the consciousness closer to subjectivity, and understanding how our consciousness works regarding consciousness research.

Consciousness Research in Science

The topic of consciousness is considered to be the most important **current scientific challenge**[112] as well as a disturbance or nuisance for science[67:27]. In neuroscience, consciousness is a continuous flow that is only accessible to the individual who experiences it, and this subjective character is among one of the greatest obstacles to methodological analysis, hence the scientific limitation in studying it.

For scientist Dean Radin from the Institute of Noetic Sciences, in California, USA, who has been studying psychic phenomena for over 40 years, **neuroscience** today sees consciousness as being generated by brain activity, however, he points out that psychic phenomena transcend these limits:

> "This suggests that the only way the mind can gain information about the world is through the conventional senses, which are assumed to be constrained by the classical boundaries of space and time. Psi phenomena indicate that the mind can transcend these boundaries and gain information without regard to constraints of space or time. Psi thus strongly challenges the prevailing neuroscience view."[113:329]

The different **scientific paradigms** interfere in research that addresses consciousness, including in the area of health. The great development of statistical techniques in the late 1940's relegated research methods that seemed too closely linked to the influences of the individual psyche to the background[114].

Behavioral science as a discipline also contributed to the marginalization of the academic study of consciousness. As a result, it has taken almost a century of development to become scientifically acceptable. Dean Radin points out that consciousness has become a **popular subject** in universities around the world. However, psychic phenomena are still very challenging for academia:

> "The conventional neuroscience perspective, which is uncritically assumed to be correct by the majority of scientists, views consciousness through the lens of the mainstream scientific worldview. That worldview regards reality as purely nihilistic, as meaningless and purposeless. From that perspective, consciousness too is therefore meaningless."[113:331.]

For Dean Radin[113], this is the predominant paradigm in science today, and as such it is being strongly defended by mainstream scientific research. Meanwhile, an alternative worldview, which considers consciousness as fundamental, is probably more correct, but definitely not a part of mainstream science. A growing number of scientists and scholars are beginning to understand that the **dominant worldview** is limited and are slowly beginning to view these alternative worldviews as more attractive.

This change illustrates the wearing out of **reductionist explanations** on science and suggests that there be an expansion of the conception of rationality accepted today, which for some researchers indicates the emergence of a new philosophical and scientific paradigm for physical, biological and human-social systems[21].

Studies based on other worldviews can be developed from different paradigms, methodologies and methods. Regardless of the choices, it is necessary to consider that the essential nature of **methodological rigor** consists in the coherence between its main elements: the paradigm that guides the research, the methodology of choice and the methods used for its development[115].

The **prevailing paradigms** in western thinking are positivism, interpretivism and critical theory. In the first, the phenomena are studied objectively and observation is the main strategy to generate knowledge and confirm hypotheses. This is the most widely used model to guide research in biomedicine and in the traditional perspective of neuroscience. In the second, science is built by assigning meaning to phenomena in an intersubjective way. The researcher's role consists in understanding and describing the meanings attributed to the concrete experiences had by people. In the third paradigm, studies are developed to bring about changes of social interest and therefore must be integrated into practice. It is up to the researcher to seek awareness of themselves and the other research participants, which requires a comprehensive understanding and analysis of the real situation, so that alternative ways of dealing with problems and their respective equations can be identified[115].

While realists advocate a material world that exists independently of observers, idealists argue that the world essentially exists in our minds. These different ways of perceiving the world influence the researchers' choice of **research methods**, in the first case, quantitative and in the second, qualitative. By perceiving this epistemological relationship, one can understand the philosophical problem by trying to combine realism/positivism with constructivism/interpretivism[90].

Some **research formats,** especially qualitative ones, make it possible to study the consciousness, such as phenomenology, by exploring the essence of the consciousness from within itself[116]; critical theory, by criticizing and trying to modify society; feminism, by questioning social roles[90]; oral history by understanding the subjectivity of the individual[114], hermeneutics, in proposing the fusion of horizons through dialogue[117], conscientiology, by focusing the object of study on the self-researching conscious being, among others.

Since the last century, biology, psychology and sociology have taken over the **psyche** as an object of study, including dreams, the unconscious and subjectivity. Although the subjective is understood as untranslatable sensations, it is typical of the individual to try to understand them and to pass on to others what they understood, hence the need to refine how scientific instruments work to succeed. With this refinement, it is possible to offer knowledge and technology for people to optimize their health and develop from their own experience.

Other areas of knowledge also propose to study the consciousness and its manifestations, based on different paradigms. Among these areas is **Conscientiology**, which focuses on consciousness research and invites the various branches of science to promote research on what is considered invisible, intangible and even absurd. It is composed of volunteers, teachers, students and researchers, and produces leading edge relative truths (verpons) based on the consciential paradigm.

Conscientiological research encourages researchers to develop critical thinking about the subjective and indissociable, by proposing a way of doing science for themselves and about themselves (self-research), for everyone and for the benefit of the Cosmos.

Consciousness Research in Conscientiology

The **neoscience conscientiology** defines the consciousness as an integral personality, beyond the limits of the human person, including, *parapsychism*, that is, the extrasensory perceptions transcending the human senses. In the conscientiological approach, the consciousness is studied considering the period before its rebirth in this human life and the experiences following the discarding of the human body or biological death[65].

According to Vieira[67:22], conscientiology's proposer, the Newtonian-Cartesian-mechanistic paradigm keeps scientists in profound and systematic **ignorance** regarding parapsychism, interdimensionality and the reality of the consciousness. Due to this limitation, science *cannot answer the whys* asked by the consciousness regarding the understanding of their own complex personality.

The scientific approach to **parapsychism,** as proposed by conscientiology, is not the same as the four other realities, from which it needs to be distinguished: occultism or popular group autism, inappropriate commercialism, sensationalism and shrewd mystification[67:24].

From the conscientiological perspective, **subjectivity** is inherent to science, because objectivity is powerless to study subjective knowledge[67:15]. And, even when studying the objective, it is the researcher who subjectively decides whether or not to accept the objective evidence in scientific findings. However, the myth of scientific neutrality extends beyond the researcher's subjectivity, by recognizing the influences it produces, through its energies, in the observed experiment.

Science, when mature, is based on the cosmoethical freedom of both its **purpose**, in terms of the use and application of the knowledge produced, and its means, in relation to the methods and honesty of the research[67:25]. Immature science, on the other hand, evades having a purpose, being satisfied with appreciating the applied method, often after compartmentalizing the researched object to the point of blocking the vision as to its totality.

The limitations of Western science favored the paradigmatic crisis and the flourishing of new paradigms, which somehow peacefully coexist with the traditional paradigm[67:28]. In this context, the best thing is to go beyond it, and provide for the **integration** of conventional science with the consciential paradigm, by which the simplest theory capable of explaining the phenomena experienced is preferred.

Vieira[1:1137] understood that, for most people who are still very much involved within the postulates of conventional, Newtonian-Cartesian, physicalist science, based on electrons and matter, conscientiology is considered pseudoscience. Thus, Vieira[1:738] recognized himself as a micro-minority in civil and scientific society. However, nowadays, countless consciousnesses already develop interparadigmatic research or approach the Thought Style of conscientiology, mixing conscientiological principles with conventional science in various nuances and, based on **personal experience**, are developing their self-research and expanding their self-awareness.

In the early 20th century, the Polish physician and biologist Ludwik **Fleck**, stated that all scientific knowledge is mutable, historical and collective. By applying the concepts of Fleck[108] to conscientiology, it is possible to recognize that Vieira, in proposing the neoscience, triggered a new Thought Style dedicated to studying the consciousness, according to the consciential paradigm.

Vieira constructed **neologisms** to define new scientific terms and to differentiate them from similar concepts that already exist, but which differ from the proposed terms. This action is in line with the proposal of Fleck[108], which guides the creation of new concepts to describe ideas that go beyond those previously defined by another collective.

He also promoted the organization of a Thought Collective of **volunteers**, acting as teachers, students and researchers. These volunteers are distributed across more than 20 *Conscientiocentric*

Institutions (CIs), with each one dedicated to researching and disseminating different conscientiological subject areas or specialties. Information on existing CIs can be accessed from the Union of International Conscientiocentric Institutions – UNICIN website, available at https://unicin.org/en/ and from the Interassistantial Services for the Internationalization of Conscientiology – ISIC website, available at https://www.isicons.org/.

Each group of people who voluntarily compose the various CIs differs slightly in a Thought Collective (TC) of their own, by bringing together researchers, students and technical support personnel to collectively think about the production and regulation of a Thought Style (TS). The same is true of the invisible colleges, research groups and conscientiocentric companies, organized on the basis of **volunteering**, who also produce and deepen the knowledge of conscientiology.

A person belongs, as noted by Fleck[108], to several Thought Collectives at the same time. When considering the **multidimensional reality,** the amount of TSs and TCs associated with this person increase even more, due to the multiple human lives accumulated, interspersed with intermissive periods, which make up the *personal holobiography*.

An opportunity to identify the TS and TC of the consciousness are the **Intermissive Courses** offered between human lives. According to researcher Tathiana Mota[118: ch.1], an

> "Intermissive Course is an advanced educational model composed of disciplines from the most diverse areas. Didactically organized according to the student's needs and delivered during the period of intermission, the purpose is to clarify the multidimensional reality of the consciousness and apply tools for evolutionary acceleration, with the aim of laying the groundwork for the next human life".

In these courses, the consciousness is invited to confront their own **holobiography**, with the opportunity to review their manifestations and concepts, and to broaden their self-awareness.

Thus, when considering extraphysical reality, one can begin to understand intermissive consciousnesses, who took an **Intermissive** Course before being reborn, as a Thought Collective with a style that includes the Principle of Disbelief, multidimensionality, interassistance and cosmoethics.

During the current life, previous TSs may be recalled and updated by the consciousness, or remain latent. Similarly, the interpersonal relationships of a collective from the past, can be revived in the present existence. The affinities promoted in Thought Collectives allow the lucid consciousness to assist their groups from the past, qualified as *groupkarma*, **evolutionary group** or evolutionary family.

The knowledge accumulated by the consciousness, life after life, composes the set of its memories, being called ***holo*memory.** Didactically, such knowledge is broken down into *cons*, or hypothetical units of lucidity. The lucidity regarding the TSs and TCs experienced in the past, through the recovery of *cons* registered in the holomemory, makes it easier for the self-researcher to avoid unnecessary repetition of their experiences, opening space for new self-cognitions and boosting their self-evolution.

The recovery of ***cons*** therefore helps the consciousness to achieve prophylaxis of the *ancestor of oneself* condition, which characterizes that consciousness who lives, today, "unconsciously repeating everything already done and surpassed in several previous human lives (seriexology), through inconvenient, counterproductive and *unnecessary self-mimicries* regarding their own consciential evolution"119[Translation].

This consciousness can compose various aspects of human knowledge, including scientific knowledge, contributing to the sacralization of theories, jettisoning science and themselves from any renewal. The consciousness thus loses the opportunity to recycle their intimate concepts, that is, to perform **intraconsciential and group recycling.**

If the Thought Collective to which this consciousness belongs moves forward in their ideas, and the consciousness excludes themselves from the group for not admitting these changes, then they experience a minor **dissidence** or *mini*dissidence in relation to the group in question. Having a notion of the unknown, the impossible, and the never are units of measurement of the consciousness' evolutionary level[75:107].

A well-known example of this mini-dissidence was described by Vieira[75:436] as the **Swedenborg Syndrome,** which relates the shift from a scientific to a religious approach by the Swedish scientist, philosopher and parapsychic Emmanuel Swedenborg (1688–1772), after experiencing a clairvoyant experience. In contrast, there is the person who recycles their knowledge to the point of breaking the bonds with their Thought Collective, experiencing a greater dissidence from their evolutionary group, or *maxi*dissidence, as reported by former Catholic priest Marcelo da Luz[120], in his book: Where does religion end?

In this context, every self-research is independent and interdependent, that is, in addition to personal motivation, the participatory *para*scientist has other intraphysical and extraphysical consciousnesses as *staff* or a work team for the sake of personal maturation[121].

Thus, one can expand Fleck's concept[108] and consider a thought *para*collective that influences the development of a *para-*

style. Thus, an important contribution of conscientiology to the theory of Fleck[108] is its recognition of multidimensional reality. This recognition will define the origin of the consciousness and its baggage of knowledge beyond this life, extrapolating the mesology and genetics to reach the paragenetics.

The conception of an idea or thought also expands and starts to compose the **thosene,** the inseparable set of thoughts-sentiments-energies. The practical effect is energy, imbued with thoughts and sentiments, that is exchanged between consciousnesses, generating a practical influence beyond the mental sphere of ideas.

Fleck[108:49] already admitted the inseparability of thought and emotion, that is, "the concept of thought absolutely free of emotions is meaningless. There is no free state of emotion in the same way that there is no pure rationality". However, Fleck needed to consider multidimensionality to complete the conception of the thosene, and to understand that the set of thosenes or **holothosenes** can influence the consciousness' actions, in most cases unconsciously, in synergy with the influence of the TS.

The application of the Principle of Disbelief by the consciousness invites the practice of transposing the Thought Style of conscientiology and of questioning the Thought Styles with which the consciousness identifies. Such an action aims to break the frontiers of knowledge in search of new leading-edge relative truths, or **verpons.**

Among the various techniques proposed for this purpose is the **consciential tabula rasa** technique, which aims to eliminate, for a whole day, conditionings, sociocultural repressions, sacralization, superstitions and brainwashings in the analysis of everything that surrounds the person. Didactically, it suggests that the person consider that they are a non-terrestrial consciousness, who just arrived on this planet for a day[75:521].

This technique presents a complex exercise of separating the individual's Thought Style that is part of a collective in their **analysis of reality**. If one's style is the way of seeing, understanding, and conceiving a body of knowledge, the first step is to recognize which style guides a person's values and decisions.

The techniques and **experiments** offered by conscientiology can help people and their respective TCs to see beyond their own TS. Such an understanding of different styles is necessary because it incorporates experiences and other strategies to understand the evolution of knowledge and the human being itself.

In this process, **disagreement** facilitates the advancement and evolution of knowledge, grounded in the verification of truths that are always changing[121]. Ambivalence, mental flexibility and avoidance of the split between right or wrong allow for the periodic review of the personal belief system and progress in self-research, because, even though scientific renewal, described by Fleck, is a collective phenomenon, it has similarities with the recycling of the consciousness. In both contexts, the saturation of disastrous experiences overwhelms pleasant ones, causing crisis, disruption and transition to a new reality, whether it is a scientific or consciential one.

Thus, conscientiological tools can help change the TS, a fundamental process for the **development of knowledge** to occur, both in science and in the consciousness. For Fleck[108], the model of knowledge production emerges from the interactionist perspective between subject and object, and reveals the dialectical conception of truth. For conscientiology, this model expands and integrates multidimensionality.

The researcher scientist of conscientiology is dedicated to the search for essential and always relative priority truths of the consciousness, manifesting as an integral human personality[67:30]. Supported by the consciential paradigm, the researcher employs some **principles** to guide their research, which are in clear opposition to the traditional scientific model, and may have similarities to social and qualitative research models. Listed below are 11 principles scientists should consider while developing their research:

1. **Cosmoethics**, in opposition to putting the means before the ends of research.

2. **Cosmovision**, in opposition to the scientific partition of research.

3. **Evolutionary intelligence**, by prioritizing research *at the core* of consciential evolution, in opposition to valuing issues that are collateral or surrounding the consciousness.

4. **Evolutionary prioritization**, in opposition to the predominantly financial motivation of research.

5. **Intellectual freedom** in acting as an independent researcher, in opposition to the institutionalization of research and dependence on funding[122].

6. **Multidimensionality**, with the experience of manifesting in multiple dimensions, in opposition to the exclusivity of intraphysicality.

7. **Parapsychism**, in opposition to the supremacy of physical equipment, instruments and tools applied in research.

8. **Participatory research**, in opposition to the myth of scientific neutrality.

9. **Self-experimentation**, based on applying the Principle of Disbelief, in opposition to fallacies and the sacralization of science.

10. **Subjectivity**, in opposition to the scientific requirement of objectivity and the replication of findings.

11. **Volunteer bonds**, in opposition to employment bonds.

In the consciential paradigm, each individual can approach their personal experiences objectively, including parapsychic phenomena and altered states of consciousness. Techniques can be used to maintain and expand a person's lucidity in an entirely natural way, without any external inducements, such as substances or body movements. Thus, the **objectivity of research** becomes possible from the experiences of one's own consciousness.

Consciential self-experimentation is a fundamental characteristic of the conscientiological scientific method, which has four fundamental elements[123]:

1. The Principle of Disbelief as a theoretical and practical supporting element.

2. Secular self-parapsychism as a logical premise.

3. Non-alignment of the bodies as the main research technique.

4. Self-evolution as a normative principle.

The daily experience of self-research makes the consciousness the greatest guinea pig of themselves, in any situation, context or location, thereby constituting their **laboratory of consciential research** (*labcon*). As a result, the researcher of conscientiology applies at least three priority scientific procedures in daily life, presented below in chronological order[67:32]:

1. Self-organization of their personal, intraphysical and extraphysical life through personal discipline.

2. Intraphysical self-experimentation of the facts and multidimensional self-experimentation of parafacts that are experienced in consciential dimensions.

3. Fixation of the evolutionary research findings in human life through the publication of verpons.

The organized experience of the researcher favors self-experimentation, the organization of findings and their publication, expanding the *corpus* of the already materialized science of conscientiology in this dimension. The main **publications** written in Conscientiology, existing at the time of preparing this book (2021), are listed below:

1. Books published by the conscientiological publisher Editares are available at www.editares.org.br. The *website* offers various books in a digital format for free, including in English. Free English-language books on this subject are also available for download at www.isicons.org.

2. Books published by the conscientiological publisher Epígrafe, available at www.epigrafe.com.br.

3. Scientific journals, listed on the Cognopolitan Institute of Geography and Statistics (ICGE) website, available at http://www.icge.org.br.

   3.1. Conscienciologia Aplicada [Applied Conscientiology], free access available at arace.org/revista-cap-consciencio-logia-aplicada.

   3.2. *Conscientia,* free access available at http://www.ceaec.org/index.php/conscientia.

   3.3. *Conscientiotherapia,* free access available at www.oic.org.br/revista-conscientiotherapia.

   3.4. Estado Mundial [World State], printed copy available for purchase at www.epigrafe.com.br.

   3.5. *Glasnost,* free access available at conscius.org.br/glasnost/index.php/glasnost.

   3.6. Holotecologia [Holothecology], printed copy available for purchase at www.epigrafe.com.br.

   3.7. *Homo Projector,* printed copy available for purchase at www.iipc.org/produto/homo-projector/.

3.8. Intercâmbio [Exchange], free access available at www.
icge.org.br/?page_id=2921.

3.9. International Journal of Conscientiology, free access
available at https://ijc.isicons.org/ijc/index.php/ijc/index.

3.10. Interparadigmas, free access available at http://www.interparadigmas.org.br (offers articles in English as well).

3.11. *Neologus,* printed copy available for purchase at www.epigrafe.com.br.

3.12. Proexologia [Proexology], free access available at apex-internacional.org/revista/index.php/proexologia/issue/archive.

3.13. Revista de Parapedagogia [Parapedagogy Journal], free access available at reaprendentia.org/pt-br/revista-de-parapedagogia.

3.14. *Scriptor,* free access available at www.icge.org.br/?page_id=2744.

3.15. Enciclopédia da Conscienciologia [Encyclopedia of Conscientiology] entries, available for free access at http://encyclossapiens.space/buscaverbete/.

In addition to written materials, there is a vast array of **free content** available on various YouTube channels, homepages and social media from institutions dedicated to the study of conscientiology. To those interested in studying and deepening this knowledge, we wish you great studies and *let's get started.*

Have you noticed a *relationship between your health* and *the expression* of your ***personal essence***? Have you noticed these relationships in people around you, whether they are colleagues or patients? Does the ***care*** *you practice and offer* on a daily basis *consider the relationship between* **health and the consciousness**?

PART II

Development of Care Practices

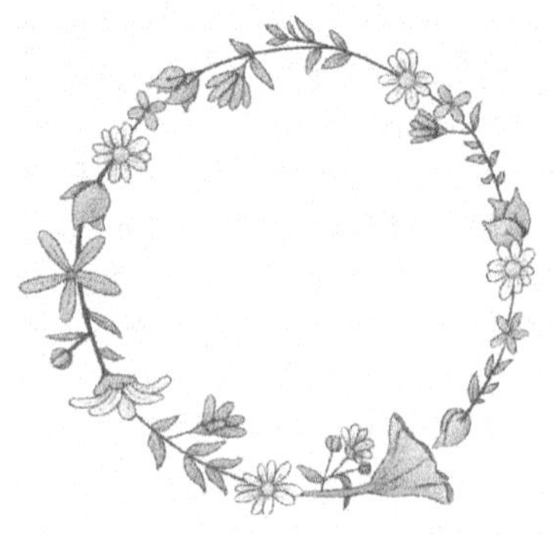

Chapter 6
Integrative Health Care

"Hurry up and live well and think that
each day is a life in itself"
Seneca (4 BC–65)

Maybe you provide a *health service.* If not, you've probably already used a service, such as a *hospital, primary care unit,* or *clinic.* How have these experiences been? What do you expect to occur in these environments? The objectives of this chapter are to understand how **health and care models** *impact integrative health care* and promote the use of *light technologies,* such as *embracement, empathy* and *interprofessional collaboration.*

Models are theoretical constructions to help understand reality. In the case of health, there are numerous proposed models involving different practices and paradigms, for example, the biomedical model, the sanitary model and the health surveillance model. These models, in addition to being theoretical, are also the government's political response to the health needs of the population[124], and accompany the changes that have occurred in the development of humanity.

The last century was marked by the **hegemony** of the biomedical model. However, this model is not homogeneous. It allows for alternatives in diagnostic and treatment practices, and for the development of movements of groups of professionals and patients who adapt and propose breaks in traditional behavior.

The influence of the biomedical model appears, for example, when people seek health services only when they are sick or in need of **immediate care**. Since the focus of these services is on complaints and health problems, it is difficult for the population to understand abstract concepts such as health promotion and disease prevention, and their aggravations. In clinical practice, the challenge of promoting health is perceived when the patient does not undergo preventive exams or screening for diseases, while, in their daily life, have trouble relating their lifestyle with risks to their health.

Due to the influence of the **biomedical model**, many health professionals focus their efforts on providing disease-centered care. But currently, health systems have received incentives from both international and national organizations to focus efforts toward integrative health care[125] that is able to meet the patient's health needs throughout their life. In order to reorient the object of health, nowadays centered around disease, beyond the patient and their complaints, it is necessary to understand the historical process of developing practices and the way that health is performed.

This need is especially present in situations where a **cure** is no longer possible, due to degenerative, progressive or incurable diseases. In these situations, palliative care that aims to alleviate the patient's suffering and improve their quality of life is adopted. The construction of integrative health care demands considering the person that is being cared for as a whole, considering their wishes and desires, and their family, articulated with the actions prescribed by the health team.

Healing, treating and controlling thus become limited postures, since these practices presuppose a static, individualized and objectifying relationship of people under health interventions. The practice of **care**, on the other hand, is not only restricted to the skills and technical tasks typical of the work process, as for Professor Ricardo Ayres:

> "More than dealing with an object, the technical intervention is truly articulated with the practice of care when the sense of intervention becomes not only the achievement of a health state sought beforehand, nor only the mechanical application of the technologies available to achieve this state, but the examination of the relationship between purposes and means, and its practical meaning for the patient, according to a dialogue as symmetrical as possible between professional and patient"[126:64,65][Translation].

Thus, the health work process, which expresses the practice and dynamic exercised by professionals and experienced by patients, can be the strategic "place" of change, provided that it invites reflection and recovers the **ethics** of a commitment to life, which includes developing a welcoming attitude, establishing bonds, seeking resoluteness and creating autonomy for patients[127].

These actions, which also characterize **humanizing** practices, can be understood as technologies to be applied in integrative health care, which are not restricted to the relationship established between the health team, the patient and their family. Similarly, the structure and organization of services should include these technologies, such as visual resources with accessible language that facilitate the movement of people within the service network, and referrals that promote access to professionals whenever necessary, in order to respond to the demands of the population.

The health worker context is relational, **dynamic** and is rich in meaning, knowledge, actions and information that need to be systematized to develop care practices. This learning and knowledge are the main asset for designing new or old technological options to improve health care practices[128].

In this sense, it is understood that technological development in health care is a process by which new, more productive and more effective means of work are created through the application of scientific knowledge, which should also include human skills, such as empathy and openness. **Technology** must not be associated only with "hard" scientific-technological development, the production of machines, equipment and instruments. The subjective aspects of the relationship established between the patient and the health care team need to walk together with the objective work process in which they interact[129].

Health Technologies

Health technology can be understood as a "set of **knowledge** and instruments that express, in service production processes, the social relations network in which its agents articulate their practice in a social totality"[129:32][Translation]. It is understood, therefore, that there is no technology outside the work process, and only within it, including both its technical and social dimensions.

From this perspective, **health work** can be divided into two types: live work in action, which refers to the work that occurs during the interaction of the health professional with the patient, as during the anamnesis (medical history) and physical examination; and dead work, which are the products means, tools and raw materials, such as an X-ray machine and a stethoscope, which the professional uses when necessary[127].

Live work in action is divided into three levels, represented through an allegory, which describes the existence of three technological toolboxes or valises used in the encounter between a health professional and a patient[130,131]:

1. **Hard**. The first valise is connected to the professional's hand and carries equipment. It symbolizes hard technology, which includes the use of machines, norms and organizational structures in each working environment.

2. **Light-hard**. The second is connected to your head and carries knowledge and expertise. It symbolizes light-hard technology, which is the specific knowledge of each professional, such as nursing, occupational therapy and psychology.

3. **Light**. The third is present in the relational space between worker and patient and includes bonding and embracing relationships, established between professionals and patients or between workers. It symbolizes light technologies that promote the **encounter** between the patient and their world of needs, as an expression of *their way of living life*, allowing health professionals to capture and make that world the object of work.

In the history of health care, different valises have already assumed a prominent position, thus defining different models of health care and the necessary skills for each health worker. For example, in the last century, the **focus** of health workers was to identify infectious and contagious diseases, and eliminate their causes (viruses, bacteria, microorganisms), strengthening the one-way health-disease model. However, with greater control of infectious diseases and the rise of chronic diseases, the multi-cause models of health-disease have gained prominence, resuming the need to consider different approaches to promote health and care, considering physical-psychic-social-environmental aspects[132].

From 1950 onwards, criticism in the field of health care grew, contrary to the large production of hard technology for medicine, related to equipment and machinery, to the detriment of light technologies, such as bonding and embracing[6]. The appreciation for hard technology caused a **distancing** from the integral view of the person in health practices and services and influenced the search for alternative and complementary treatments in the late 20th century.

The body as the focus of care, promoted by predominantly hard technologies, remains under investigation. In a study conducted by Gonçalves[129] with physicians and nurses from health centers in the city of São Paulo, it was common for these professionals to have difficulty in directly indicating an **object of work**, in addition to the patient's body and individual care. In this case, the professionals did not fully recognize the patient as an object of care, focusing on the immediate biological demands of their specialty.

This difficulty may be related to the **appreciation** of the technical nature of health practices, to the detriment of the social nature, which would consider economic, political, ideological, biological and cultural conditions. Recomposing the patient's integrality requires reconceptualizing the object of these practices, and building new relationships in different fields of health care[133].

To reinforce this view, Gonçalves[129] considers the **complexity** of health technology, since

> "the work process is not just a mechanical expenditure of forces: it is the most human form of sociality, of historical genesis.

> In each grain of technology, all the determinants of the past and all the living constructions of the future are simultaneously contained"[129:268][Translation].

At every meeting in the world of health care, one must invest in the production and **defense of the life** of the other, without repeating the privatization of care, which occurs when the professional takes possession of the patient's autonomy when deliberating on their daily care. The exclusion of patients from participating in this construction occurs, for example, by making them say what the professional wishes to hear, based on practices of control about the other's way of life[131].

To overcome the hegemonic model, it is necessary to restore a practice of **liberating** care, organize work processes that are increasingly shared, and follow a person-centered logic. This allows for the daily construction of close bonds and commitments between workers and patients in technological health interventions, according to individual and collective needs[131].

Health work does not have a fully structured object, and its action technologies are configured in processes of active **intervention**, operating with technologies of relationships and encounters of subjectivities. Therefore, it goes beyond structured technological knowledge and involves a significant degree of freedom in choosing the way to carry out this production of health care[131].

Thinking about an **anti-hegemonic model** capable of making the micro-decision dynamic more public, captured by the world of people's needs, is not simple. The current fragmentation of the health sector, in specific population groups, hampers projects that would invest in health as a public good, as a patrimony of the whole society and are of inestimable individual and collective value[131].

In this process, it is necessary to promote light technology in health, expressed as a process of producing *interceding* relationships, which is not a sum of one with the other, but a **meeting space** for their intersections. It is configured, for example, through the embracing, empowering and bonding practices[131].

A survey that accompanied medical consultations showed that physicians usually interrupt patients after 11 seconds of **conversation**. As a result, the chances of physicians identifying specific aspects that are important to the patient to be addressed in the clinical encounter, are reduced [134].

Health care is made up of workers from different professional groups, who together are able to respond to a wide range of health **needs**. Teamwork, therefore, is an opportunity to improve Primary Health Care responsiveness, given the increase in the number of health disciplines and its possibilities of care actions, and the scarcity of human resources, especially physicians; which can also prevent the fragmentation of health care[135,136].

Therefore, over the last decade, teamwork has been approached under the logic of **collaboration**, with an emphasis on the following attributes: interdependence of professional actions, concentration on the needs of health service patients, negotiation between professionals, shared decision-making, mutual respect and trust among professionals, and recognition of the role and work of different professional groups[137].

Teamwork seeks to expand access and **coverage** of the population served, but it also responds to the need for an integration of disciplines and professions, understood as essential for the development of health practices, based on the new biopsychosocial conception of the health-disease process. It increasingly emphasizes the health team as a productive unit instead of the independent and isolated work of each individual professional separately[111].

Teamwork can be defined as the collective contribution of professionals to **decision-making**, with a focus on solving problems to achieve the best performance, where everyone shares goals and is collectively responsible for the results[138].

However, the biomedical model may result not only in the **fragmentation** of care when treating the patient, but also in the fragmentation that occurs in relations between health professionals in which each one just takes care of their domain, with no communication between professionals, or between professionals and patients, with the latter, being the most interested in care[139].

Another definition describes teamwork as a daily practice triggered by the needs of the patient and involves integration, trust, respect, availability for collaboration, a sense of belonging, humility, and time to listen and talk. This practice requires **communication** skills and sharing of the workspace to ensure frequent contact and sociability, the appreciation and familiarity of different professional practices and roles, especially in complex cases, and shared leadership to deal with conflicts and tensions[137]. From this perspective, the following recommendations can be adopted to improve the teamwork of health professionals:

1. Promote interprofessional communication;

2. Understand that teamwork is a daily practice and involves integration, synergy, availability and reliability;

3. Invest in the efforts to know the roles and responsibilities of the different team members;

4. Understand that interprofessional conflicts interfere with teamwork in primary health care;

5. Understand that teamwork depends on a network of reference and counter-reference;

6. Consider that working conditions interfere with teamwork;

7. Assume that the goal of teamwork is to respond to health needs.

WHO defines **collaborative practice** in the field of health as the actions of health professionals from different areas who provide services with respect to the integrality of health care, while involving patients and their family, caregivers and the community, in order to provide high quality care at all levels[140].

A Brazilian group of nurses[141] deepened the discussion on interprofessional collaboration regarding the concept of **person-centered care**, and presents the following three key elements:

1. The principle of integrality in the expanded perspective of health care, understood as a response to the health needs of patients, families and communities.

2. Empowerment, autonomy and user participation in the provision of care.

3. The professional-patient relationship, based on effective and open communication, in a flow of information and knowledge exchange, in order to contemplate the expression of the patient's subjectivity and autonomy.

Understanding the essential elements for collaborative teamwork promotes the creation of an educational, professional qualification and reference **network** that can overcome the fragmentation of the biomedical paradigm.

In this sense, it is worth highlighting other practices that also promote **integrative health care,** such as complementary therapies and humanizing practices, which include such characteristics as a focus on people, considering their social and family contexts; broad and holistic approaches; valuing non-biomedical knowledge and practices that address multiple forms of care; encouragement of self-healing, active participation and empowerment of patients; a family and community approach[102].

These characteristics are not exclusive to any health and care model or practice, and can even be found in the professional practice offered within the biomedical model. The practice of consciential health also promotes these characteristics, based on the **consciential paradigm**.

Consciential Health Practice

Assistantial techniques directly or indirectly promote the improvement of the person's consciential health. These techniques act in four phases synthesized in the polynomial: **welcoming–clarification–referral–follow-up**, proposed by Professor Waldo Vieira for the experience of interassistantiality[1:76].

Personal qualification to help other consciousnesses begins, therefore, in the quality of your personal welcoming or **embracing**. Without this first step, every skill you gain becomes ineffective to help others. That is why it is important to deepen the understanding of this condition, which we will treat here as universal embracement.

Universal embracement is defined as "the posture, position, or condition of the lucid, conciliatory and fraternal conscin in assistantially receiving other intra or extraphysical consciousnesses, granting resolutive attention, sustained by their self-orthothosenation and principles of cosmoethics"[142][Translation].

Orthothosenity expresses the quality of healthy and cosmoethical thoughts, sentiments and energies with correct intentions that characterizes the assisting professional at the moment of embracement. This condition prevents the distortion of goals and the deviation of interests in the care practice. Acquiring and sustaining universal embracement involves[142]:

1. the act of knowing how to live in an assistantial manner;
2. fraternal self-prioritization;
3. assistantial self-availability;
4. support in coping with problems;
5. helping others to acquire autonomy;
6. group cooperation;
7. the search for the individual's uniqueness;
8. the development of potentialities;
9. clarifying interassistance;
10. the anti-conflictive life;
11. cosmoethical selflessness;
12. a universalist sense;
13. consciential openness;
14. cosmovision;
15. the coexistence of help and mutual respect.

Universal embracement can be achieved through energetic, parapsychic and cosmoethical self-qualification, with the aim of attending the integral demands of consciousnesses. It also proposes the experience of multidimensionality in joint action with the extraphysical helper's team[142]. The **collation** of the main facilitators and obstacles faced by the consciousness interested in developing universal embracement is described in the following table:

Table 2. Comparison of facilitators and hinderers of universal embracement[142].

No	Facilitators	Hinderers
1	Empathy	Apathy
2	Energetic self-control	Energetic decompensation
3	Enhanced listening	Inattentive listening
4	Evolutionary conviviality	Selfish conviviality
5	Gratitude	Misunderstanding
6	Healthy habits	Addictions
7	Orthothosene	Pathothosene
8	Proactivity	Defensiveness
9	Protagonism	Victimization
10	Responsibility	Guilt
11	Secrecy	Gossip
12	Serenity	Hastiness
13	Very rare friendship	Idle friendship

Embracement implies **understanding** the health paradigm experienced by the other, to support them within their own recognized universe, and to invite them to broaden their vision. Such an attitude demands accepting the reality of the other, as it is, to initiate the connection. The acceptance of the reality of others requires the professional's interest and openness to new ideas, in order to subsequently carry out the interpolation of possible knowledge with the assisted person. Thus, acceptance becomes the synthesis of the embracing.

From this moment on, the professional comes closer to the paradigm of the assisted person with possible **therapeutic** approaches. In this way, it will facilitate the transformation of the patient's paradigm, at the same time that the paradigm of the professional will also be transformed, when faced with new world perspectives.

In the end, the professional will return to their own paradigm, which they consider most legitimate and coherent for themselves, with some degree of personal **change**. They end up being, therefore, the most assisted or benefited by the assistance provided, and by the opportunity to transform and evolve.

Within embracement, a space is established for the **clarification** of the other, considering their needs and interests. Here, it is worth mentioning two types of assistantial tasks: the assistantial task of clarification, or claritask, and the assistantial task of consolation, or consoltask. The claritask is more complex, demands clarification, assisting the other in learning and expanding their personal knowledge. The consoltask is less complex, meets more basic needs, such as hunger, thirst or the momentary consolation of personal anxiety, without addressing the therapy needed for the assisted person to achieve self-overcoming.

Based on the popular expression that it is better to teach a person how to fish than to give them a fish, whenever possible, it is better to **prioritize** clarification, which promotes greater autonomy and long-term sustainability. However, both tasks have their place in the assistantial process and are determined by the needs of the person being assisted. In many cases, the consoltask precedes the claritask, providing the minimal structure for the other person to think for themselves, and being essential for the claritask to come.

It is important to recall that clarification occurs in an interaction between consciousnesses, when the assisted person accesses information that helps them to think and **reflect freely**, either through conventional dialogue, or from the energies, attitudes, or thoughts of the assisting professional.

The construction of a space for thinking freely, without indoctrination and gurulatry, is carried out at all times by consciousnesses that work in the care environment, based on personal **intentions**. Embracement and clarification begin to fail when there is an interest in enticing, indoctrinating, dogmatizing or convincing the person by force[1:87]. The Principle of Disbelief, taken to its ultimate cosmoethical consequence, results in prophylaxis against interpersonal manipulations.

After clarification, the process continues with the **referral** or prescription of necessary actions to support the decisions made by the assisted person, for example, through five actions listed below:

1. Inclusion of new therapies, either self or heteroconducted, to support the personal changes sought.

2. Articulating with other professionals involved in the therapy, who are already participating or still to be included.

3. Dialogue and mediation of conflicts with other people involved, such as family and friends.

4. Energetic support by the professional and extraphysical helper's team.

5. Conducting unhealthy extraphysical consciousnesses involved in the problem, for extraphysical treatment, reducing the unbalanced interaction between them and the person.

The referral phase occurs with greater or lesser assistance from the assisting person, depending on the degree of autonomy of the assisted person. Here, the principle of encouraging consciential **self-sufficiency** is again valid.

In the end, the **follow-up** of the assisted person allows the assisting professional to observe the development of the assistance provided. This is when the professional identifies new action points to help the assisted person, allowing for new interventions. The professional deepens their understanding of the immediate and mediate effects of the assistantial process, broadening their systemic view or cosmovision. And they also consolidate their understanding in terms of their ability to provide assistance, promoting renewals in themselves and adopting those skills already developed and demonstrated during the assistance. Follow-up is the moment of actual feedback, when the assisting professional is invited to reflect on the effects of the assistance provided.

Monitoring is not always easy, and it may even be contrary to the choice of the person being assisted, when opting for isolation. Physical distances and even busy routines are other complicating factors. In this context, lucid cosmoethical parapsychism is a unique **resource** for enabling access to the development of the assistance performed and for analyzing the insights inspired by the extraphysical helpers.

The separation of interassistance into four phases is didactic, and the intention is not to reduce or simplify it. In practice, each assistantial context is unique, and it includes elements of the phases presented, to compose the whole evolutionary **history** of the consciousnesses involved.

The application of resources and techniques derived from conscientiology for the treatment of the consciousness' diseases and paradiseases is studied by the conscientiological specialty called **con-**

scientiotherapy[q]. Its practice can be conducted by the consciousness themselves, or it can be supported by conscientiotherapists from the International Organization of Conscientiotherapy – OIC.

It is worth recalling that consciential health is not intended to be an exclusive matter for conscientiology volunteers and researchers. Our wish is that, just as other care approaches are being made available in health services, this book inspires readers to **incorporate** the techniques proposed by conscientiology into their own self-care practice and in the practices applied by professionals. In this way, readers contribute to the development of self-awareness, evolutionary conviviality and health practices.

As a health care professional, which *health and care* **models** *influence your health and care* **practices**? As a patient, how do you *perceive this* **influence** on the dynamic approach of health services and in the *assistance provided*?

---

q https://en.oic.org.br/consciencioterapia

Chapter 7
Co-development of Care

Now that we have expanded the models of health and care, and the concept of health technologies, how do you *apply the different valises* in your health practices? How much do these practices allow for listening and pondering together with the patient for the *co-development of care actions*? The objective of this chapter is to deepen the person's understanding regarding the integrality **of health care** and their **autonomy**, based on an understanding of the amplified clinic, the anti-protocol, the unique therapeutic project, and the case study of pain and multidimensional care.

Identifying technology in the health area as an intentional know-how, mediated by reflection, reason and human experiences, allows professionals to rediscover their **autonomous, responsible, reflective, coherent identity** and consider subjectivity for an integrated, singular and scientific practice, that is, a technological practice[128].

However, this is not a simple process, as each **professional** has different instruments, content and attitudes in their health practice, including or not including complementary therapies, humanizing practices or conscientiological techniques.

In the case of Western medicine, the professional presents knowledge and expertise that were developed within classical physics and the fragmentation of the organism. Thus, it will be a **challenge** for this professional to include a light technology that is not part of this framework[143].

An example of this situation is the current difficulty in including **integrality** within the health practice. The theory of Western medicine, linked to scientific knowledge, was not built within an integral framework, and it has been very difficult to modify the practice, since this knowledge dominates the cognitive and therapeutic action of hegemonic biomedical professionals[143].

Each medical rationale presents different knowledge and reveals how these influences the health practice. All interpretative and **therapeutic** processes will be restricted and directed by the values, methods and stylistic limits, and all knowledge and action in health and disease will be more or less complete, extensive and truthful in consistency with the respective conceptions and characteristics of the rationales[143].

Therefore, the rationales that already understand man as an integral being in his **cosmology** facilitate this approach in diagnosis and therapy. However, this is not always the case, for example, in situations where homeopathic medicines are used alone or when acupuncture is treated as just another commercialized specialty[143].

Traditional Chinese medicine, as a medical rationale, presents, in its cosmology, an integral view of the human being that facilitates the practice within this perception of **care**. Homeopathy also presents, both in knowledge and in practice, a higher level of integrality. Thus, the insertion of these rationales and "what they offer to the population in the area of Primary Health Care is a promising strategy for enriching and expanding the coefficient of integrality in practices"[143:204][Translation].

Primary Health Care provides the best conditions for the use of these technologies within the health care services network, because, compared to the hospital, it is less historically committed to the culture of biomedical specialties and also offers space for greatest amount of autonomy for both professionals and patients[7,143].

In order to facilitate access to different rationales, it is essential to train **hybrid professionals**, who, by knowing about complementary therapies and different health practices, are able to put the patient's therapeutic project in the foreground and consider the risks and benefits together to choose the best therapeutic path at each moment[6]. From this perspective,

> "It is possible that a physician, nurse or physiotherapist knows at least basic acupuncture procedures for the most frequent problems, which will lead them, for example, to practice auriculotherapy by inserting mustard seeds at specific points in the patients' ear, without initially acting with all their rational potential, but certainly expanding the traditional clinic"[40:151][Translation].

Sometimes, this professional may have had access to the entire theory of rationality in traditional Chinese medicine, or they may simply be using an isolated technique to extend the treatment. In any case, it is questioned whether the fact of using such practices from other rationales would already be **sufficient** to expand the clinic.

By using an isolated auriculotherapy practice, this professional would be expanding the therapeutic options offered. But would they also be **expanding** the applied health model? If yes, this action would be helping the patient become more aware of their health process; if not, they would simply be proposing a different technique, which the patient would accept, even without increasing their autonomy and integrality in their health-oriented self-care.

The introduction of other rationales should be carried out to **improve** the relationship between professionals and patients, and to make the most of the integrality, autonomy and self-care frameworks of these practices. However, these premises are not always achieved in practice.

Often, the reasoning and terminology of different rationalities can be quite confusing for the lay public, causing **estrangement** from both professionals and patients with these practices. Terms such as *Yin* and *Yang*, *Similia similibus curantur*, *Vata*, *Pita* and *Kapha*, common in traditional Chinese medicine, homeopathy and ayurvedic medicine, are some examples commonly used to explain diagnoses and therapies.

Integrating complementary therapies pose risks and requires understanding the inherent **limitations** of each medical rationale, therefore

> "all medicines and cultures have limits in their treatment of the health-disease process, in their efficacy/effectiveness/veracity, both in health promotion and in the diagnosis and prevention of illnesses and therapies. It is these limits that make the issue of integrality relevant and of public interest, regardless of the medical rationale analyzed"[143:202][Translation].

In addition to integrality, incorporating **autonomy** in health care is also a challenge for various rationales, besides Western medicine, since the professional can offer complementary therapies without providing humanized care, or being committed to the patient and their lifestyle. In this way, the professional continues to exercise a fragmented practice, even though offering complementary therapies.

However, articulating actions of integrality and autonomy with structured knowledge (whether clinical, epidemiological or representative of other health care models) is essential in health establishments to **produce** access, embracement, bonding, accountability, resoluteness and effectiveness, commitment and empowerment of patients, given the different *ways of living life*[131].

In this way, if technology is not just the application of science or simply a way of doing it, but a **decision** about what things can and should be done. Healthcare professionals should think about how they are mediating and choosing what they should want, be and do to those they assist and to themselves[126].

Thus, for complementary therapies and humanizing practices to be present, it is not only necessary to broaden the scientific bases of technologies beyond the biomedical sciences, but also to work towards **reconstructing** the intersubjective interactions of care, through listening, embracing and empathizing, in order for the presence of the other, the individual under care, to be more effective and creative[126].

The proposal is to decrease the focus of the individual's care from an external perspective, while developing this outlook from within the person, permeated by a relationship of bonding and embracement. But without falling into the common place of **"biopower"**, expressed by Foucault[144], which occurs when the person is given freedom to care for themselves, but there is only one right way to do it: the one proposed by the health team. During clinical practice, how does the professional react when the patient's care decision goes against their technical recommendation, beliefs and personal choices?

One aspect that can **transform** a therapeutic encounter into a care relationship is the possibility of relating the technical aspect to the human aspects of care, in order to overcome the individualistic conformation of the health conception as a "complete well-being" that is immutable and isolated from people's life experience[126].

It has already been demonstrated that the incorporation of other rationales and practices can enrich Western medicine toward the **recovery** of human aspects of care. It has also been shown that the provision and incorporation of light technologies are desirable resources for this process. However, neither patients nor professionals usually know how to manage these resources satisfactorily, perhaps because of their lack of meaning and significance for the daily life of the other[126].

Thus, professionals are expected to approach theory with practice in this process of personal development, while promoting autonomy and proactivity that is capable of increasing their understanding of themselves and others. This non-transferable process can have a ripple effect, encouraging others to also follow this path as a result of **therapeutic exemplarism**, where everyone ultimately benefits.

In Primary Health Care, this situation becomes a real issue, for example, when professionals and patients are surprised by the lack of **results** when mechanically fulfilling their roles, procedures and protocols, guided by a clinical-preventive logic of risk control and functional normality[40,126].

Alternative practices that reflect the meaning behind the use of these technologies, such as the **appreciation** of *practical wisdom* or *phronesis*[126], the Antiprotocol movement[40] and the amplified clinic seek to rekindle in professionals and patients the practice of technological and humanized care.

Practical wisdom[126] shows how the recognition and revaluation of the human being's project of happiness establishes a bridge between the meaning of existence and issues more directly related to their experience and care in health, reflecting positively on ways of acting and interacting in human relationships in health practices.

Also, in this proposal of clinical qualification and work co-management, physician and researcher Gustavo Tenório Cunha[40] proposed the **Antiprotocol**, which went against the idea of valuing the biological aspect of the sick subject, and assumptions of the simplicity and immutability of reality, resulting in a lack of responsibility for the professionals.

Antiprotocol is a management approach fully developed for Primary Health Care, which can also be understood as a **team working method**. It consists of three movements: use of indicators to perform an analysis of the situation and diagnosis, choice of possible resources and assimilation of the guidelines for the Amplified Clinic[40].

The Amplified Clinic's guidelines include increasing the autonomy of the person, family and community by increasing resources to provide for their health. From this viewpoint, and based on reports of the common habits of Primary Health Care teams, Cunha[40] presents **suggestions** for improving treatment success:

1. Avoid pastoral and blaming recommendations.

2. Reinforce that a multifactorial disease has no single cause.

3. Negotiate restrictions without rancor and take into account the patient's investments.

4. Work with offers, not just restrictions.

5. Specify offers for each person.

6. Avoid initiating queries by questioning affertions and behaviors.

7. Value the quality of life.

8. Ask what the patient understood about what was said about their illness and medication.

9. Avoid saying "always" or "never" (preferring the concept of possibilities).

10. Avoid frightening the patient.

11. Remember that chronic illness cannot be the only concern in life.

12. Balance fighting the disease with production in life.

13. Avoid the medicalization of life, that is, don't medicalize normal situations of human existence, such as mourning, adolescence and aging, by transforming them into clinical situations.

14. Act in morbid events with a maximum level of support and a minimum level of medication.

15. Prefer phytotherapy to diazepines whenever possible.

Although these recommendations are presented within an integrative panorama, the author chose to organize antiprotocols for diseases in order to facilitate the incorporation of these **guidelines** by the health team, which is hegemonically formed in the biomedical tradition. As an example, we can mention is the Antiprotocol for Smoking, which highlights the importance of team meetings, preparation of the Singular Therapeutic Project (STP), and the organization of home visits[40].

The STP is an **action plan** developed jointly between the health team and service network and the patient and their family and community, to meet the current and future health needs of the patient, based on the definition of goals, actions and responsibilities to monitor and reassess the co-development of care[145].

The Amplified Clinic concept and the STP proposal invites one to understand that the situations described by the professional team as '**difficult** to understand' are often cases that come up against the limits of traditional clinical practice. In these cases, the suggestion is to perform an extended anamnesis (medical history), with the intention of helping the team to enrich the meetings based on the voice of the patients[40].

The **extended anamnesis** aims to listen to the patient, based on their ideas and words, without much direction and without doubting facts that theories do not explain, except in cases of urgent healthcare. Cunha[40] cites as an example of this situation an account from a patient who claimed that "*it only hurts when it rains*", and explains:

> "A more complete clinical history, without filters, has a therapeutic function in itself, since it situates the symptoms in the sick person's life and gives them the opportunity to speak, which implies some degree of analysis about the situation itself. In addition, this anamnesis allows professionals to recognize the individual's uniqueness and the limits of diagnostic classifications, in order to recognize the patient beyond their diabetes or hypertension"[40:190,191][Translation].

In addition, other rationales present, in their paradigm, a **reference** that allows one to relate rain to pain. For example, in traditional Chinese medicine, the theory of five movements considers the excess of "humidity" in the body, which is influenced by the humidity of the environment, and is a determinant in diagnosis and therapy.

Knowledge of the existence and understanding of other rationales, provided to professionals by complementary therapies, prepares them for the **multiplicity** of realities they will face. Conversely, restriction to any health practice will limit their provision of care.

It is necessary to highlight the property of **extended listening** for clinical practice. Usually, there are patients who, just by being listened to, feel better or more confident to face the disease. Listening without judgment or analysis, and understanding what the person feels and who they are, by itself, enables them to change for the better[146].

To illustrate this reality, we have retrieved the story of the medical resident who, faced with an intense work routine, when reporting the case of a patient who got sick while walking with his dog, was surprised by his tutor question: **what was the dog's name?** At this point, the resident reports that he did not understand the question, but follows the suggestion. After asking the patient and talking for a few minutes about the dog, he noticed that a change began to occur. At the time, the resident did not know how to measure the effect of this change, but, over time, reports that the ability to see the other beyond the disease had an effect on himself and on the care that was provided[147].

Therefore, it is important to expand the anamnesis and clinical practice with knowledge of other rationales and practices, provided that they are carried out with respect to the **human aspects of care**, which involves embracing the other's worldview, connecting with the person's integral being and autonomy to guide their own life.

Based on a perception of the person's complexity, the need for a **leading** role in the project of care is clear. That is, in addition to prescribing and guiding actions, health professionals need to hear what is important to the patient, and what their limits and difficulties are, based on some essential aspects[40]:

1. Try to find out the meaning of the disease for the patient (why do you think you got sick?).

2. Ask how the patient feels about the disease (how do the problems affect your life?).

3. Get to know the singularities of the person (fears, angers, manias and temperament, sleep and dreams).

4. Assess whether there is denial of the disease, what is the capacity for autonomy and possible secondary gains from the disease.

5. Identify what feelings the professional develops for the patient during the meetings, and the limits and possibilities for the clinical relationship.

6. Get to know about the patient's projects and dreams (wishes) and leisure activities (present and past).

"These are questions that in a very reasonable number of times point to paths, if not towards the therapeutic project, at least towards the deepening of the bond with and understanding of the subject"[40:194][Translation], besides important **questions** to improve one's understanding about the meaning and application of light technologies.

Logically, one understands that it is difficult to achieve this whole approach with the growing **demand** of patients and the reduced time available to attend them. However, it is not necessary to obtain all this information during the first contact, nor to overload professionals in their activities. These are questions to encourage professionals to practice creative and committed care, not only with patients, but also with the professionals themselves, recognized as supporting characters of this change[40].

Returning to *practical wisdom*, it is possible to trace other important **converging** points of change for professionals in relation to their clinical practice. The case of Mrs. Violet reported by the physician Ricardo Ayres[126] exemplifies this change.

Mrs. Violet is a lady with uncontrolled hypertension who always arrived at the physician's office complaining about how long things took and how much time she had already spent waiting. In one of the visits, the physician, instead of disregarding this complaint and focusing on the disease's progression, invited the patient to speak about herself. Based on this humanized approach, the consultations became meetings. In this case, the physician speaks about how the change of his attitude toward the patient promoted the recovery of her existential project and allowed him to establish an effective therapeutic bond and health management actions that made sense to her, resulting in more autonomous control of her living conditions[148].

This case is able to greatly exemplify how an expanded or complex approach to the person allows us to explore different results that go beyond the repetition of attitudes that result in problems in the professionals' practice. With this, it continues the search for **achieving** a truly humanized practice that is satisfactory to professionals and patients.

It also retrieves the **purpose** of health, and by extension, of life itself, without which the motivation for self-care becomes meaningless. The very etiology of the illnesses that affect the patient can originate from the absence of goals in life, and its resulting self-realization. The perception of a mobilizing purpose and even the delineation of a meaning for life are therapeutic in themselves.

The presence of *practical wisdom* in the case of Mrs. Violet, was identified as the **differential** that made the humanization movement and the transformation of care in this therapeutic encounter possible [126]. "The provision of care as a designation of health care that is immediately interested in the existential meaning of the experience regarding the physical or mental illness, and therefore also of health promotion, protection or recovery practices" [126:89][Translation].

The difference in the meeting described between the professional and the user was the **opening** of an authentic interest in listening to the other. This ability to listen and establish dialogue is related to a technological device that is essential to the human aspect of care: embracement. Without becoming confused between the reception/welcoming center, this device is present in the continuous interaction between patients and health services[126].

Instead of simply avoiding the **noise** that was primarily detected in the interaction, the professional and the patient improved their dialogue and thus assumed co-responsibility for the provision of care in the therapeutic relationship. A bonding relationship was built, which was necessary for the commitment of each one to their own actions[126].

As a result of this health care, professionals and patients continually rebuild care in a responsible **feedback** loop. It is also possible to expect an enrichment of therapeutic possibilities beyond the body and its functioning, promoting reflection on the ethical, moral and political meanings of health practices[126].

The Case of Pain

Let's take a very common complaint in health care as an example, for the reconstruction of care: pain. The concept of pain in the biomedical paradigm is the unpleasant feeling or emotional

experience associated with actual or potential tissue damage. Acute pain is characterized by lasting less than 30 days; and chronic pain longer than 30 days[149]. Chronic pain affects between 30 to 50% of the world population. In Brazil, 39% of the population lives with chronic pain[150]. In the United States, 30% of the population reports chronic pain. Pain can be classified into three types[149]:

1. **Nociceptive:** triggered by the physiological activation of pain receptors, related to bone, muscle or ligament tissue injury. It generally responds well to symptomatic treatment with analgesics or non-steroidal anti-inflammatory drugs (NSAIDs).

2. **Neuropathic:** resulting from injury or dysfunction of the nervous system or abnormal activation of the pain pathway. It responds poorly to common analgesics (paracetamol, dipyrone, NSAIDs and weak opioids).

3. **Mixed:** related to the compression of nerves and roots that generate neuropathic pain and musculoskeletal structures (bones, joints, ligaments) that generate nociceptive pain.

In addition to this classification, there is fibromyalgia (extensive chronic pain associated with multiple symptoms, such as fatigue, sleep disorder, cognitive dysfunction and depressive episodes) and myofascial pain (presence of trigger points distributed along vulnerable muscles), which are treated separately due to their **complexity**[149].

The **treatment** of nociceptive and mixed pain must comply with the World Health Organization's proposal of scaling, consisting of the steps of the analgesic ladder, which progressively uses analgesic drugs, NSAIDs, adjuvant drugs and opioids (weak and strong) in a progressive way. The basis for neuropathic pain treatment involves the use of tricyclic antidepressants and antiepileptic drugs in most cases, with opioids being reserved only for patients with refractory pain to antidepressants[149].

From this perspective, most pain treatment in the biomedical paradigm involves staggered **medication** which, although very efficient, shows difficulties in its use, as listed below[149]:

1. Abandonment of treatment due to adverse effects (between 20 and 30% of patients).

2. A lack of advantages in using antidepressants when compared to a placebo, in the treatment of nonspecific lower back pain or repetitive strain pain in the arm.

3. No evidence of benefits from the use of opioids, regardless of their potency, over a prolonged period of time for patients with nociceptive pain (such as osteoarthritis, rheumatoid arthritis and lower back pain, among other diseases).

4. A relationship between tramadol and an increased risk of suicide.

5. Even with the indication of opioids for cancer pain, in some cases, patients have difficulties in pain management.

6. Patients complaining of chronic pain frequently suffer from depression, which should be promptly treated.

Thus, to achieve better results in pain treatment, some recommendations are beginning to **appear** in the scientific literature[149]:

1. Most patients with nociceptive pain and fibromyalgia benefit from regular physical exercise.

2. Cognitive-behavioral therapy, massage, rehabilitation and locally applied heat are effective alternatives to treating muscle or nociceptive pain.

3. There is no effective drug treatment for fibromyalgia, just regular physical activity and the treatment of comorbidities such as anxiety and depression.

4. Regular physical activity, cognitive-behavioral therapy, local heat therapy or physiotherapy can be used by patients with all types of pain (nociceptive, neuropathic or mixed) depending on the patient's physical capacity and under the supervision of a qualified professional.

5. Acupuncture and diazepam are equally effective in treating acute pain in osteoarthritis.

6. In cases of myofascial pain, in addition to drug treatment, the practice of acupuncture and dry needling on trigger points is effective, in addition to regular physical activity.

7. The practice of acupuncture is beneficial in the treatment of osteoarthritis and chronic muscle pain.

8. In the case of chronic muscle pain, common analgesics and NSAIDs are indicated only when chronic pain is acute and not as a maintenance treatment.

In 2003, WHO produced a report with more than 100 indications for the use of **acupuncture,** based on an analysis of clinical trials. In relation to analgesia, acupuncture promotes pain relief between 55 and 85% of patients. It might even be higher when compared to powerful drugs such as morphine, which achieves 70% relief; and much higher than the placebo effect, which provides relief to only 30 to 35% of patients. The illnesses indicated by WHO for treatment with acupuncture, which are directly related to pain, are listed below in alphabetical order[151]:

1. acute epigastric pain (in peptic ulcer, acute and chronic gastritis, and gastrospasm);

2. adverse reactions to radiotherapy and/or chemotherapy;

3. biliary colic;

4. cervical pain;

5. depression (including depressive neurosis and depression after stroke);

6. dysentery;

7. facial pain (including craniomandibular disorders);

8. headache;

9. knee pain;

10. lower back pain;

11. nausea and vomiting;

12. pain in dentistry (including dental pain and temporomandibular disorder);

13. periarthritis of the shoulder;

14. primary dysmenorrhea;

15. postoperative pain;

16. renal colic;

17. rheumatoid arthritis;

18. sciatica;

19. sprains;

20. tennis elbow.

Thus, the **progress** of pain treatment beyond medication is observed, including other practices and recommendations. Moreover, each medical rationale or health practice has a way of understanding pain, relating it to its biological and psychic meaning.

The proposal, therefore, in the case of pain and health-disease processes with which it is related, is to focus one's attention beyond the body, to understand what it may **symbolically** be "telling us".

For Dr. Ryke Geerd Hamer, real or imaginary conflicts can trigger illnesses that are actually part of "biological survival programs" made to face different threats and dangers, perceived consciously or unconscious by the patient[152].

Considering the unconscious component of illnesses, it is often easier to access emotions through the **body** than by conscious awareness expressed through verbal language, as the body functions as a more direct physical portal to the emotional brain and often is far more powerful than thought or verbal language[53:33]. The role of professionals and patients in this context is to promote connection and, depending on the case, reflection, understanding and accountability, but without blame.

Therefore, when considering the **approach** to pain based on different medical rationales and health practices, it is essential to do so in the context of humanized care, supported by embracement that develops qualified listening, a bond that reveals life projects, and actions in health that values the autonomy and creativity of the health team and the patients.

Multidimensional Care

From the perspective of multidimensional care, the interaction between the caregiver and the patient promotes a change in the patient's holothosene for the better. The intentional mobilization of consciential energies and the patient's immersion in the caregiver's holothosene enhances the **therapeutic performance**, beyond the available biomedical techniques and resources[1:522].

In this context, it is worthwhile for the health professional to qualify their control of **consciential energies** and personal thosenity, to be applied in the care of others. The consciential paradigm, for example, offers several techniques composed of technology that is available to professionals and to those who are interested, in order to boost the development potential for interassistance. The daily experience of these techniques, especially the Vibrational State (VS), *sympathetic assimilation* (symas), and *sympathetic deassimilation* (symdeas) of consciential energies, extends the therapeutic environment beyond the professional performance in clinics and hospitals, based on the positive energy of the caregiver wherever they are.

Thus, the VS becomes a **therapeutic key** for care[1], as it goes beyond the professional's need for energetic balance, and is concretely applied to the therapy itself, whether in the energizing of medications and dressings, in the direct mobilization of the patient's energies, or by interaction with the caregiver's healthy holothosene.

On the other hand, the non-application of bioenergetic techniques predisposes the caregiver to professional **energetic intoxication,** from the energies of different environments and consciousnesses, whether or not these professionals admit the bioenergetic dimension[75:427]. This intoxication results from the natural process of interaction between the caregiver's energies with the patient, the different environments, and teams in which they work, due to the interfusion of energies present in each exchanged look, word, feeling and thosene. The deepening energetic interfusion, commonly promoted by the caregiver during the therapeutic act, characterizes the *sympathetic assimilation* (symas) of consciential energies. At this moment, parapsychic awareness and energetic scanning may even lead the therapist to feel what the patient emotionally or physically feels. Energetic intoxication is a contributing yet under explored factor that makes up the multiple causes of burnout syndrome.

Burnout syndrome is typically characterized by three dimensions: emotional exhaustion, dehumanization (or depersonalization), and reduced professional achievement. Emotional exhaustion, in turn, is characterized by mental and physical exhaustion and a feeling of incapacity, which can lead to symptoms of anxiety and depression. The consequence (and cause) of this condition is dehumanization, which is a state in which the person becomes indifferent, impersonal, ironic and cynical toward others, as a form of social distancing and in an attempt to minimize exhaustion. Finally, the activities performed lose their meaning and the individual experiences a feeling of failure and dissatisfaction[153].

Burnout can have implications that range from the personal sphere, with more serious consequences such as the abuse of psychoactive substances and suicide, to the professional and collective spheres, which can result in risk to the patients themselves. Among the main **physical consequences** of burnout are excessive fatigue, sleep disorders, muscle pain, headaches, gastrointestinal disorders, eating disorders and reduced immunity. Cognitive signs and symptoms can include difficulty concentrating, memory impairment and slow thinking; emotional signs are irritation, anxiety, depression, discouragement and aggressiveness; and behavioral factors include inhibition, neglect, loss of initiative, tendency to isolation, lack of interest in work and/or leisure and lack of flexibility[153].

Understanding the energetic intoxications inherent in the caregiver's actions is then essential to prevent burnout and its cascading effects on one's own, family and social health. The reversal of this trend is to achieve interassistantial **solidarity** between the caregiver, the patient and their family.

Intoxication, even though it may predominantly occur during therapeutic practices, often occurs at other times of the day, due to the fraternal and welcoming **holothosene** of the caregiver, who is available to assist others in any situation.

This holothosene, associated with the principles of cosmoethics and the consciential paradigm, when applied to care practices, characterizes the multidimensional caregiver[153]. In addition to health technologies, it is used in the consciential paradigm to perform bioenergetic scanning, deintrusion and facilitate the patient's reeducation and recycling[153], by applying, for example, ten **multidimensional practices** listed below:

1. **VS.** Perform the prophylactic vibrational state.

2. **Parapsychic signal.** Consider your personal energetic and parapsychic signals, which express signs and sensations arising from extrasensory perceptions, to guide assistance.

3. **Symas.** Perform the assimilation and deassimilation of your consciential energies during consultations.

4. **Bait.** Promote lucid baiting of the sick extraphysical consciousness, drawing it close to yourself, the caregiver, and allowing it to be assisted by your healthy holothosene.

5. **Parapsychism.** Apply lucid parapsychism for the benefit of intraphysical and extraphysical patients.

6. **Projection.** Understand the multidimensional reality of the patient from the extraphysical dimension, through the use of lucid projection.

7. **Penta.** Continue assisting in the personal energetic task (penta), from the daily donation of healthy energies, and consider clarifying suggestions transmitted by the extraphyscal helper during the task about the best way to approach and treat the assisted person.

8. **Offiex.** Use the advanced resource of the extraphysical workshop (offiex), achieved with the veteran practice of penta.

9. **Recin.** Seek self-reflection leading to recycling self-change in the assisting and assisted person.

10. **Post-desoma**. Promote the post-desomatic reception after biological death and continue to assist the patient in the extraphysical dimension.

The adoption of the multidimensional reality facilitates the caregiver to recover their innate knowledge, prior to this life, enabling them to experience the ten **conditions** listed below[153]:

1. **Benevolence:** development of heterobeneficence.

2. **Claritask:** clarification for consciential pro-autonomy.

3. **Symdeas:** personal effectiveness in energetic deassimilation.

4. **Skills:** resuming innate assistantial potential.

5. **Opportunity:** recovery of lost assistantial opportunities.

6. **Parapsychism:** identification of parapsychic phenomena.

7. **Proexis:** a view of the proexis in decision-making.

8. **Recovery:** regaining the health and well-being of the bedridden person.

9. **Re-education:** persistent self-commitment to your consciential evolution.

10. **Responsibilities:** cosmoethical self-responsibility.

Another perspective of multidimensional care is when the patient brings their own parapsychic experiences into the **therapeutic encounter** that directly impact their health.

When the interaction with **parapsychic phenomena** is not understood by the person who experiences it, it usually brings anguish and suffering, due to the simple ignorance of the real meaning behind these sensations. Noticing this difference within themselves, and having emotions and sensations that do not fit into the experienced paradigm, leads the person to conclude that the *problem is theirs*, and not a limitation of the paradigm in which they live by. It is common for a person not to share these sensations with anyone, assuming that it is *some sort of madness*, which increases their suffering even further. In these cases, an expansion of the paradigm by adding the multidimensional reality is the first step towards a healthier interaction with themselves. Understanding the benign character of one's sensations de-dramatizes the problem and allows one to focus on improving one's relationship with the multidimensionality.

The cinema is full of good examples on how this conflict of paradigms occurs, especially when the situation involves **post-desomatic parapsychosis**, which is when the consciex is unaware that they are no longer a conscin manifesting in the human dimension. After physical death, the consciousness continues to perceive themselves as *alive,* thinking and interacting, and, supported by their personal beliefs, concludes that they are alive in this human dimension. The table below provides three examples of films with this theme:

Table 3. Examples of parapsychic experiences and phenomena in the cinema.

Film	Experience	Phenomenon
The Sixth Sense (1999)	It portrays the conflict experienced by the character Cole Sear (Haley Joel Asment), who has visions of dead people walking among the living, and is assisted by his therapist (Bruce Willis) to interact with these consciexes and provide help and comfort to them.	At the same time as guiding the patient, the therapist himself is helped to understand that he himself was a consciex, who had already passed through physical death, and was experiencing post-desomatic parapsychosis.
The Others (2001)	In the film it's *the living who torment the dead* when Grace's (Nicole Kidman) family begins to experience strange phenomena in the house where she lives, with curtains and doors opening without reason. Such phenomena are actually produced by the conscins who also inhabit the house.	Grace and her family are actually consciexes, in a parapsychotic condition, who did not know that they had already passed through physical death, but this understanding is not enough to help them overcome this condition. In the end, it is the living who decide to leave the house, because Grace and her family cannot admit their own condition.
A Simple Formality (1994)	The famous writer Onoff (Gérard Depardieu) is interrogated by the police inspector (Roman Polanski) at the police station during a murder investigation after having been found in the vicinity of the crime scene. In the end, he recalls that the murder under investigation was actually his own suicide.	Initially, Onoff doesn't remember anything. Gradually, fragments of memory appear, until reaching the memory of what he had been done. The film portrays well the assembled parapsychodrama, to treat parapsychosis in the extraphysical dimension, which helps Onoff to remember his own suicide and, based on that, allows him to continue his extraphysical life.

The experience of parapsychism, however, does not shield the person from expressing associated mental illnesses. Thus, there can be a diagnosis of **mental disorder** in the person who also manifests parapsychic experiences, interacting and bringing variations in the typical expression of the disease. This fact, despite initially hampering or confusing the diagnosis, allows us to look at the person fully, based on the principle that the roots of human diseases are in the consciousness.

The film A Beautiful Mind (2001) depicts the concurrence of these syndromes. Despite historical inaccuracies, the plot is inspired by the life of American mathematician John Nash. In the plot, he is diagnosed with schizophrenia due to his recurrent delusions and hallucinations. Gradually, Nash learns to distinguish what is real from what is "imaginary", creating a more harmonious relationship with himself and his family. However, the dialogue and consistency of the same people present in his hallucinations suggest another diagnostic perspective: the moments experienced could be real interactions with extraphysical consciousnesses. By admitting this **hypothesis**, the approach and treatment could be expanded, adjusted, and meet the person's needs with greater precision.

Other manifestations of multidimensional reality can get confused or overlap with biomedical diagnoses. In this case, the risk of **medicalizing life** is expanded to the *medicalization of multidimensionality* experienced by the consciousness. Therefore, considering multiple dimensions expands the possibilities of assistance, bringing new therapeutic and meaningful perspectives within the consciential paradigm. Below are five examples of multidimensional conditions related to possible diagnoses in conventional medicine:

Table 4. Multidimensional conditions related to possible diagnoses in conventional medicine.

Western medicine	Consciential paradigm	Consciential therapy
Depression	Intraphysical melancholy (melin) due to a deviation from the proexis	Resumption of action in the existential program
Phantom pain	Perception of the psychosoma at the location of the amputated physical limb	Energetic self-control
Hallucination, delirium, psychosis	Unconscious parapsychism, parapsychic lability	Energetic self-control and development of lucid parapsychism
Recurrent nightmares, night terror	Nightmare projection, recurrent retrocognitive dreams, projective catalepsy	Energetic self-control and development of lucid parapsychism
Panic syndrome	Thanatophobia (extreme fear of death)	Multidimensional self-awareness

A common example is that of the ectoplast consciousness who, due to having a predisposition towards the densification of energies, is also more predisposed to everyday accidents with themselves, whether it is falls, stumbles, bumps, or with the objects they interact with, such as breaking glasses, burning light bulbs or crashing computers. **Ectoplasm** itself is not negative. On the contrary, it has great potential for self-evolution and assistance to other consciousnesses. What is lacking, in this case, is for the consciousness to coordinate their energies in a more harmonious way, to compensate for the excess of dense energies that they naturally manifest and that resemble pseudopods of energy that extend beyond their energosoma. One of the possible causes for confusion, in this case, is simplifying the diagnosis to a framework of inattention, hyperactivity or anxiety that may also be present, concomitantly with ectoplasm. And, if multidimensionality changes the relationship of the person with their health, health conditions can also arouse interest in multidimensionality.

Experiences related to death and illness, such as the **Near-Death Experience** (NDE), an interest in communicating with a deceased loved one, the phenomena of improvement upon death and the farewell projection can awaken in the consciousness the desire to understand the multidimensional reality.

The NDE is a **phenomenon** that has been extensively studied in science due to the volume and convergence of details in patient reports. It consists of having the experience of lucidly leaving the body at a critical moment of health, such as a serious traffic accident or surgery, in which the person is provoked to reflect on their life, and must decide whether to return to life or go through physical death. An improvement upon death occurs when the patient, usually disillusioned and about to die, suddenly improves, bringing hope to family members and less experienced professionals about their recovery, but, following this, the person dies. On the other hand, the farewell projection is the experience of the consciousness seeing or feeling the presence of a loved person at the time of their biological death, motivated by the desire of the person who is dying to say goodbye to that consciousness.

Helping another person to understand their parapsychic experiences requires that the professional be willing to give up, at some level, applying their own life paradigm, for the sake of the other person's worldview and recovery of their health. From this point on, it is possible to build **therapeutic projects** tailored to needs and interests that harmonize the dissonance between parapsychic experiences not yet understood and the person's paradigm of life, which is causing their suffering. In this process, there is a recovery of the person's purpose of life, existential values, and innate ideas that they had before being born.

It is thus intended that the role of the health professional as a multidimensional caregiver is to develop care spaces that consider the intraphysical and extraphysical dimensions, promote physical-parapsychic listening and caregiver-patient interaction within a biomedical-integrative-consciential paradigm. These spaces demand the **recycling** of workers and the work process, through the promotion of the trinomial formal education-self-teaching-permanent self-experimentation.

What amount of **autonomy** do you allow others to have, when conducting therapeutic and interassistantial practices? How much do you assume your *legitimate role* as a **co-author** in the development of your care, when in the position of patient? *Do you perceive the energetic and multidimensional interactions?* If so, what are the **effects** as a caregiver or patient?

Chapter 8
Self-care

"It is part of the cure to wish to be cured."

Seneca (4 BC–65)

What do you already do for yourself? How much do you *take control of your own* self-care? How do you integrate it into your everyday life? The objectives of this chapter are to present which factors are related to a **mature self-existence** and to propose the **FEMA method** to guide the *dynamic and continuous cycle of self-care.*

In the consciential paradigm, we are the result of three inseparable **factors**: genetics inherited from our ancestors, paragenetics inherited from ourselves and the influence of the environment around us.

In **genetics**, trends in the genetic code are encoded, which may or may not be expressed, according to the influence of other variables in the body and the surrounding environment. It is in approaching this aspect that we will list the diseases and protective factors of our parents, grandparents, siblings and relatives, food intolerances, subclinical discomforts and risk factors to be prevented. It is also the time to learn about the habits and solutions that most helped them to deal with their problems, making part of the family's traditional knowledge, passed down from generation to generation, and which in many cases is not registered in health textbooks. For example, that food intolerance to soy, identified by the mother's trial and error, and later identified in the daughter. Or that intestinal colic that improves when the father drinks lemonade, and which also relieves the child's colic when he ingests it.

In addition to family genetics, there are genetic traits that can be adopted even when a person does not know their biological family. This is the case of celiac disease, which affects white people more, and glaucoma, which affects black people more, or breast cancer, which affects women more, and obstructive sleep apnea, which affects men more. Do you know the **family genetic risks** you are subject to? What about the protective health factors inherited from your family?

In ***paragenetics***, personal tendencies expressed in this or other lives are encoded. This is when we map out the diseases, illnesses and symptoms that were important in previous lifetimes, and that led us to disability or even death. We learn the lessons from the habits already experienced and are able to minimize their occurrences. We analyze the interaction of our temperament with our health, for example, selfishness and depression, anxiety and obesity, resilience and burnout. The examples left by a previous version of ourselves allow us to apply what was learned in the past and avoid the same mistakes in the present. Are you aware of your paragenetic health risks? What did you get sick from in your past lives?

The influence of the environment, also called **mesology,** defines the interaction of the environment on our health. The spectrum of elements that make up mesology is extensive, ranging from physical aspects such as pollution and variety of food, to energetic aspects, such as the quality of the energies from different environments and the consciousnesses that surround us, to the cultural context in which we are inserted, with its predominant beliefs and paradigms. Being lucid about these influences is challenging, because we adapt to the environment to the point of not noticing it, or consider it the only possible reality. The consequence is to consider certain risks to our own health as natural, whether it be the stress of daily life, traffic pollution, or the biomedical health model we adopt.

By seeking to understand how these three aspects impact us, we transform our present-future by identifying and recycling personal traits that no longer benefit us, and assuming and strengthening traits that drive our evolution. The steps of personal change can be demonstrated in the following three **models**, in a proposed chronological order:

1. **Self-conscientiotherapeutic cycle:** self-research–self-diagnosis–self-confrontation–self-overcoming[154-156].

2. **Self-conscientiometric cycle:** evaluation-diagnosis-recycling-reevaluation[157].

3. **FEMA method of self-care:** Find-Embrace-Move-Again proposed in this chapter.

The central agent of these actions in these three models is the person who will experience the change, based on the principle that lucid consciential health begins with **self-research**. Only when a person assumes that they are the most responsible for understanding and conducting themselves do they take direction of their own life and health. At that moment, they become a *guinea-pig conscin* of themselves, an object of self-research reaching advanced consciential health, conducted in a self-aware way, with the purpose of potentiating their own evolution[69].

The guinea-pig conscin applies the Principle of Disbelief in their self-research, is assertive in the use of their bodies of manifestation and is attentive to the flow of life in the cosmos, in order to better understand their own inconsistencies and syndromes. Thus, it predisposes them to intimate **recycling**, which can be described as the elimination of wounds and the obtaining of a "holosomatic presential intelligence" in order to recompose sediments present in their psychossoma[158]. To assume one's own health is to assume evolution itself. Before that, the person will instinctively take care of their own health, remedying problems after they have already occurred. They prefer not to look for the causes of their problems, and instead believe in simplistic and miraculous solutions to recover the health that they deliberately wasted. This is the phase of the consciousness' still in primary or elementary health.

When a person becomes **lucid**, they build an understanding of what health means for them, adjusting their desires and expectations, and in many cases, reviewing the punitive concept of disease for an understanding of the disease as a dialogue with themselves and their needs.

The construction of a **personal health reference** also initiates a new relationship between the consciousness and reality, starting from the holosoma for all instances of life, and little by little producing answers to the questions:

1. What is health for me?

2. What is illness for me?

3. What is care for me?

4. What are my self-care habits related to:

   4.1. Sleep?

   4.2. Nutrition?

   4.3. Personal hygiene?

   4.4. Physical activity?

   4.5. Socializing with family and friends?

   4.6. Stress management?

   4.7. Vibrational state?

5. What is my health paradigm?

6. What rationales and practices do I adopt in my self-care:

   6.1. Western medicine?

   6.2. Traditional Chinese medicine?

   6.3. Anthroposophic medicine?

   6.4. Homeopathy?

   6.5. Ayurvedic Medicine?

   6.6. Phytotherapy?

   6.7. Osteopathy?

   6.8. Chiropractic?

   6.9. Meditation?

   6.10. Other practices?

7. What factors are involved in my health?

8. What role do I play in my self-care and what role are health professionals, family and friends expecting?

9. How much health do I need to achieve my life goals?

10. How many years do I want to live? And how will I keep my body alive until then?

11. What is the limit of my interassistantial donations in accordance with my baseline health that is necessary for maintaining life?

12. What are my main risks of illness to be prevented? And how do I prevent them?

13. What are the likely tendencies towards loss of autonomy and independence as I age? And how do I prepare for them? And how do I prepare my family and friends for them?

14. How can I prepare myself and the people around me for my death? What action do I need to take to do this?

15. What projects do I want to be continued after my death? And how can this be done?

One proposal to help build the personal health framework is to draw a **self-timeline** of health-disease-care considering all phases of life, as shown in Figure 1 below:

Figure 1. Self-timeline of health-disease-care.

Self-timeline of Health-Disease-Care

Name:

Date:

Self-reflection	Childhood	Adolescence	Adulthood	Third age	Fourth age
How would you describe your health condition in general?					
What illnesses or problems can be reported?					
What medical practices and procedures have been used?					
What were the most significant memories from that time?					
How do I see myself at this stage in my life?					

Instructions

Use this Timeline to organize information about your health condition, diseases and healthcare resources.

Try to find a connection between these stages of life based on your memory or with the help of friends and family.

Add and organize the information as needed.

This information can help you develop the different stages of the FEMA Method, considering the continuous and dynamic cycle of self-care.

Download at www.autocuidado.org/blog

Getting to know ourselves by recovering our personal biography can be an additional benefit to this process of examining our health and disease situations. Another positive effect is that based on the traced hindsight, we can build a forecast for the future. One type of practice from anthroposophic medicine is the **biographical methodology,** which may be an important ally in rethinking the life history of each person, considering the particularities and possibilities of each trajectory[159].

The perception of consciential health is increasingly expanded when exploring our own history, through identifying new signs that express the harmonious experience in all areas of life, thus predisposing self-healing, such as with these 30 **attitudes**, listed below:

1. **Active sexuality:** a harmonious affective-sexual relationship.

2. **Anti-addiction:** a life without addictions[160].

3. **Anti-conflict:** an intimate posture of seeking elements of convergence with other consciousnesses, especially those of lesser affinity, through empathy and understanding the other's reality.

4. **Anti-rubbish:** the habit of keeping only healthy belongings with you, eliminating objects that are negative, evocative or loaded with unhealthy gravitating energies, capable of harmfully influencing the environment and thosenity of consciousnesses[161,162].

5. **Assistantiality:** sincerely helping other consciousnesses, in harmony with the extraphysical helpers[163].

6. **Authenticity:** genuinely expressing yourself, without masking or manipulations[164].

7. **Cosmoethics:** personal ethics in relation to everything and every part of the cosmos.

8. **Cultivating healthy leisure:** the wisdom of spending time to gain consciential health[75:538].

9. **Energetic balance:** the frequent practice of prophylactic Vibrational States (VSs) and the sympathetic deassimilation of energies.

10. **Financial organization:** a harmonious positive relationship with money and assets.

11. **Fraternism:** a legitimate feeling of well-being for all beings[1:581].

12. **Good mood:** a healthy mood, which is positively contagious, without the negative distortions of irony and sadism. "A *good mood* is consciential health"[75:579].

13. **Healthy routines:** the daily experience of habits that build your personal proexis[165].

14. **Lucid projectability:** exciting experiences in other dimensions[166].

15. **Mental hygiene:** cultivation of a clean and organized mind, discarding and recycling what no longer serves[75:656].

16. **Neophilia:** healthy curiosity that mobilizes self-experimentation, renewal and access to leading-edge relative truths.

17. **Openness:** a personal disposition to unravelling neoideas and neorealities.

18. **Optimism:** the realistic expectation that the best possible thing will happen, for you and everyone[75:70].

19. **Orthothosenity:** the maintenance of healthy thosenity that enhances your organic immunity[75:432].

20. **Peacemaking:** a peaceful and pacifying presence[75:650].

21. **Penta:** daily interassistantial practice.

22. **Personal hygiene:** maintaining self-care of the body and mind[75:609].

23. **Personal self-motivation:** the intimate motivation and the intrinsic satisfaction of undertaking work in progress, which expresses the experience of the motivation-work-leisure trinomial.

24. **Proactivity:** intimate availability to act in favor of evolution[72].

25. **Self-confrontation:** honest dialogue with yourself, without *sugarcoating* or compromising[167].

26. **Self-discernment:** thoughtful decisions in everyday life, without anxiety or unnecessary delays[1:541].

27. **Self-disposition:** a personal willingness to accomplish your goals[1:624].

28. **Self-imperturbability:** an unshakable, positive, and frank manifestation in the face of life's contingencies[1:141].

29. **Self-incorruptibility:** incorruptibility demonstrating the health of the mentalsoma[168:412].

30. **Serenity:** a calm, tranquil and harmonious attitude in different environments and groups where you act[75:128].

The positive expression of health is contagious and instigates, in the person who witnesses these attitudes, the desire to obtain a level of health already achieved by the observed consciousness. The health signs listed above, although they may be subtle and non-quantifiable, are significant for those who live with them in their daily life. This is how the principle of **exemplarism** works, when contact with the most harmonious reality of the other predisposes the consciousness to reflect on their own interests and needs.

By deciding to achieve them, the consciousness becomes determined to carry out personal recycling and to recover the best version of themselves, in general, experienced during their most recent intermissive course. This maximum healthy expression already achieved by the consciousness represents the **homeostatic reference pattern**[169], being a feasible objective to be accessed and set in the current life.

The set of signs that express one's health forms the ideal reference, profile or consciential health model, through which the consciousness establishes **healthy goals** to be developed and achieved based on this health pattern[72].

Close observation of reality also has another effect, that being an increase in one's understanding of the health offered, marketed and disseminated in everyday life. Health is an object of **desire**, sold in beautiful packages and promising miraculous solutions to treat personal anxieties. There are so many "novelties" and contradictory information that can confuse more than help, making it difficult for you to choose the right one.

Therefore, the best way is to refine one's **cosmovision,** by continually developing an understanding of the world of health and health in the world. By broadening one's critical view of media content, one avoids being seduced by the very desire to obtain a magic solution. After all, the best seller is the buyer themselves, when they project their expectations on the product offered.

The purpose of seeing beyond is to transcend everyday news, to go beyond and gain greater autonomy in one's personal choices. In this way, the consciousness builds and applies their own method to verify the **truth** of the information that interests them, in reliable sources and with the support of experts. The protocols, guidelines, discussion groups and other excellent resources available on social networks on the internet help each consciousness to take the best evolutionary advantage for themselves and others.

A qualified perception of reality is essential for a **balanced self-relationship**, and allows the consciousness to take a stand on, for example, these 16 issues that are reported daily, reflecting an interest in their own health:

1. **Activity.** The practice of frequent physical activity.

2. **Alcohol.** Avoidance of alcohol consumption and other legal and illegal drugs.

3. **Aluminum.** The use of deodorant without aluminum.

4. **Cigarette.** Avoidance of smoking and going to places with secondhand smoke.

5. **Cured meats.** Avoidance of consuming cured meat products, high in preservatives and sodium.

6. **Drinks.** Avoidance of drinks with added sugar in your daily routine.

7. **Food.** Daily consumption of fresh food (fruits, vegetables), preferring *to peel off than unpack.*

8. **Hands.** The habit of hand washing to prevent disease transmission.

9. **Intolerance.** Recognition of personal food intolerances.

10. **Meat.** Reducing meat consumption, based on an omnivorous, plant-based or vegan diet.

11. **Mouth.** The habit of oral hygiene, with or without fluoride.

12. **Nails.** Use of the personal manicure and pedicure kit.

13. **Pesticides.** Avoidance of pesticides.

14. **Plastic.** The maximum reduction in the use of plastics with bisphenol A for consuming heated food.

15. **Sweeteners.** Avoidance of artificial sweeteners.

16. **Transgenics.** Minimizing the consumption of transgenic foods.

Self-Care Triad

Self-care are actions taken by people for the **benefit** of their life, health and well-being and that contribute to their development and aging[170]. From a consciential perspective, self-care demonstrates a mature self-relationship, based on experimentation and incorporation of healthy habits and useful routines, which increase one's personal and group harmony, thus boosting one's consciential evolution.

The desires of the consciousness directs their self-care actions in the search to close the gap between who they already are and who they want to be. However, just wanting is not enough, as reaching a new level of health depends on the practical implementation of these **actions**, supported by the three main personal powers: will, intentionality and self-organization[171].

Self-care, as a personal prophylactic-therapeutic **strategy**, favors recycling and reaching new evolutionary levels. It is the result of combining three factors that relate to and influence each other: self-knowledge (understanding oneself and the personal health framework), the cosmovision of health (a critical view of the knowledge and health technologies offered), and the good use of available health resources (techniques, practices and professionals). Self-care can thus be summarized in the following schematic representation (Figure 2), in which the elements interact as a triad.

Figure 2. Self-Care Triad.

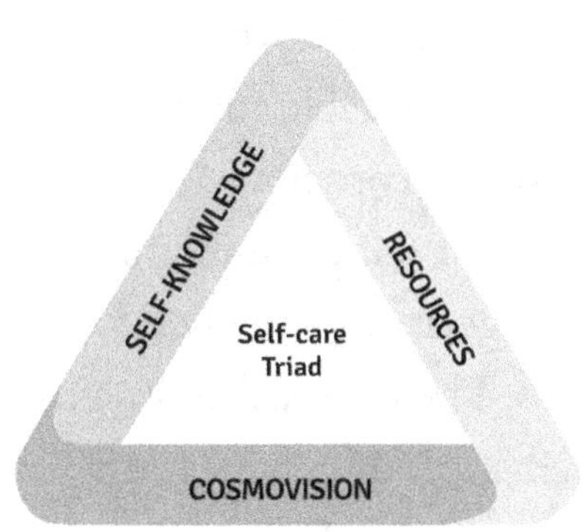

In the self-care process, the consciousness gradually refines their personal health model, their life goals, health tools and technologies, qualifying their personal valise to be applied on themselves and others. The consciousness' parapsychism also increases, allowing more psychic tools to be included in their personal valise. In this way, their research **transcends** physical reality and the time period of this life, and allows them to understand their personal and group reality from an even broader and more systemic perspective.

The identification and selection of available health resources requires research, critical analysis and experimentation. Although relevant, because they accelerate the achievement of results, they do not replace the will and determination of the consciousness, and should not be adopted as a universal panacea or the solution to all problems. No matter how good the technique, the practice or the professional, they will always be **tools** at the service of the consciousness, and will not replace their own recycling and personal efforts.

FEMA Method for Self-Care

Based on the ideas discussed so far, the FEMA method was structured to guide the dynamic and continuous **cycle** of self-care, whether from the perspective of promotion, prevention, treatment or rehabilitation, thus supporting the development of consciential health. This method is applicable for a range of conditions, from more subtle realities of the consciousness, such as discomfort, anxieties, symptoms, traits of temperament and interests, to concrete conditions already categorized by medical rationales, such as a diagnosed disease or illness. The approach is integrative and consciential, considering the interaction of genetics-paragenetics-mesology and physical-bioenergetic-emotional-mental-parapsychic perspectives.

The term **FEMA** is an acronym for the Find-Embrace-Move-Again polynomial. Like other continuous improvement practices, the method is structured in stages to facilitate its application and lucid experimentation by the interested person. However, its separation into steps is didactic, and variations may occur, for example, with concomitant steps or elements of one stage overlapping that of another, according to the dynamic of each consciousness.

The FEMA method is not restrictive and can be applied interdependently from the practices, approaches and tools existing in conscientiology and other areas of human knowledge, with a focus on the **qualification** of self-care, based on the self-scientificity–self-conscientiometry–self-conscientiotherapy–self-research polynomial[172].

The four **steps** of the FEMA method are detailed below:

I. Find

The **first** step is to find, search, identify and discover:

1) alterations, symptoms, difficulties, discomforts, grievances, anxieties, diseases, illnesses, imbalances, weaktraits (weak traits), absentraits (absent traits), thosenes that demand attention; and wants, interests, desires, strongtraits (strong traits), insights, inspirations;

2) health professionals who can help in this process, such as physicians, nurses, dentists, physiotherapists, psychologists, social workers, massage therapists, osteopaths, homeopaths, naturologists, acupuncturists, Reiki practitioners, coachs, conscientiotherapists;

3) paradigms and rationales that can guide health care, such as traditional Chinese medicine, anthroposophy, ayurveda, Western medicine, homeopathy, complementary therapies and consciential health;

4) help groups, virtual communities and people related to the same problem or interest.

The search and identification of a personal need helps the person to **explore** and recognize their own consciential reality. At this point, it is worth asking: what bothers me? What are my needs? What do I want to treat? The answers can vary from sensations to illnesses or even to new qualities desired by the person. Below are some examples of possible needs, broken down by types, to make the exercise easier to understand.

With regard to **sensations**, I can try to understand in my daily life if I feel irritated when I am upset or if I get nervous for no reason.

I can try to understand which **symptoms** cause me discomfort, for example, if I feel tightness in the chest several times a day or if I feel coolness in my right leg even thought I don't feel cold throughout the rest of my body.

As for my **thoughts**, do I think about sex more than I'd like to or do I repeatedly have thoughts that I'm a failure?

Regarding **diseases**, I can try to identify if I have any kind of eye allergy that constantly bothers me or if I'm afraid of developing a common problem in my family, such as diabetes or hypertension.

In relation to my **behavior**, do I have traits that I need to recycle, such as mental rigidity or difficulty in making decisions (decidophobia), which interfere with my family and social life, or the dispersion of attention and efforts that make it difficult for me to complete the tasks scheduled on my calendar and disorganize my routine. Moreover, do I have traits that I could improve, such as being a better listener or more generous.

I can also have **personal interests** to develop, such as a desire to improve my relationship with my brother or to master the vibrational state. Including also more deep-down issues that I want to discover about myself, which can appear as insights, such as the intimate certainty that I have something important to do in this life, although I still don't quite know what it is.

Next, it is necessary to identify the practices and professionals that will be adopted by you. It is when the consciousness asks: how do I want to **address** my need?

This step may require consultations with different specialists and the completion of questionnaires, evaluations and exams to start your self-research. Often, more than one consultation with different professionals is needed to find the right approach, leading to a journey similar to a pilgrimage among professionals. Certain diseases may even deserve a second opinion. During this process, uncertainty and frustration due to a lack of **responses** can generate anguish and the desire to give up, requiring the person to redouble their determination and persistence.

Another point of attention at this time is not to become **paralyzed** or resigned with closed diagnoses that do not invite self-research, such as hyperactivity, autoimmune disease or terminal stage illness. This invitation applies both to patients and health professionals, especially in cases where there is no longer a chance of cure in this life. The frustration of expecting a cure, combined with the idealization of health, prevents professionals from considering the provision of integrative health care, for example, using technologies such as a unique therapeutic project or starting palliative care.

The **difficulty** in offering integrative health care can be noticed in the situations reported in the cases of Lucy and Jane and in the critical case of Anthony, described below:

The case of Lucy

Migraines appeared during adolescence, always accompanied by a lot of pain and an attempt to relieve it through various treatments. Lucy had already consulted with different health professionals covered by her health insurance, tried a diet that restricted some foods, physiotherapy, massage and used strong medicines, but the pain continued. And now, how can we help Lucy? How can we find a solution to this situation?

The case of Jane

Since she was a little girl, she remembers being overweight, and was never very fond of physical activity, nor diets. Jane was accompanied by a health team at the health center, and the exams were always being amended. She had diabetes, hypertension and was morbidly obese. The guidelines were always carried out, her family had already been addressed, but the situation did not change. How could we intervene in Jane's health? What technologies could be used?

The case of Anthony

He is in the terminal stage due to pancreatic cancer and is admitted to the ICU to receive advanced care. The ICU team maintains the chemotherapy prescribed for cancer, which is now beginning to have as a side effect the loss of sensation in the hands and feet. With no prospect of cure, the damage caused by chemotherapy, at this moment, is beginning to outweigh the benefits. How long will it take for the health team to realize that chemotherapy no longer brings relevant benefits and deserves to be stopped? And, when withdrawing it, what can the ICU team offer to Anthony and his family to replace the efforts previously dedicated to the hope of a cure? What are the needs of Anthony and his family at this moment to be met by the ICU health professionals?

In addition to the health team, patients also have difficulties in seeking integrative health care. The problem can range from the concept of health, through knowledge of existing therapeutic alternatives and practices, to the moment of looking for a professional who brings together the desired qualities. When **choosing** a professional, five resources can help you to make the best decision, as listed below:

1. Their membership to professional associations and institutes dedicated to the subject in question, as informed by the lists of accredited or associated members available on websites. Being affiliated with a society does not guarantee competence, but demonstrates the interest and dedication of the professional in qualifying for the subject matter. For example, the accredited physiotherapist at the Mackenzie Institute or the Spine Doctor associated with the corresponding medical association.

2. Their professional qualifications or *curriculum vitae*, when available on clinical websites, personal webpages and social media. Through their résumé, it is possible to understand the main topics of interest, experience and scientific production of the professional.

3. Articles, speeches and videos made by the professional available in electronic magazines and on websites, blogs and social media. It is an excellent tool to understand the professional's Thought Style and language, allowing one to identify affinities in the health care approach.

4. Customer reviews posted on *professional's search sites* and across the internet.

5. Indications and reports of experiences made by groups of people with similar needs, who meet in person or through social networks.

This stage may also require extra **costs**, so check the therapeutic possibilities in your neighborhood, public services available in your region, services linked to universities, popular clinics, and also recommendations from colleagues and family members.

A free and potentially effective resource is help **groups**, virtual communities, and people connected to the similar problem or interest. To participate in groups is to learn from the experience of others, optimizing your self-care efforts.

When choosing a medical rationale, it is still common for people to seek a biomedical practice and, only when the improvement goals are not met, do they start to consider a so-called new complementary therapy or alternative practice. This model relegates non-biomedical practices to a second stage in treatment, reducing its value. However, it is worth reversing this **logic**, and to assume integrative health care from the beginning, including practices of all types in the treatment, according to your desires and needs.

There are **limitations** to all the approaches that deserve to be considered when making a choice. Medicine is not very efficient in diagnosing and treating disorders that do not fit a diagnosis, either because the symptoms are mild, subliminal, with an incomplete expression; or when they require the integration of multiple specialties. Still, many insist on settling for biomedical limitations rather than broadening their gaze to "unconventional" options.

II. Embrace

The second stage invites people to understand, comprehend and **embrace** changes, symptoms, discomforts, diseases, insights and desires, without judgments or blame, in order to understand yourself and foster self-care. Embracement involves cosmoethics, gratitude, compassion and forgiveness.

The challenge at this moment is to integrate the **discomfort** experienced in yourself, making it a part of your essence, as opposed to considering it a *disturbing external entity*. Embracing a problem redirects the energies which were previously dedicated to avoiding it, in an effort to work on its solution. Embracing makes it easy to think and plan solutions. Initially, embracing occurs without one understanding the intimate reasons that have contributed to triggering that disease; whether the reasons are conflicts, desires or needs.

Sometimes we can be seeking knowledge of the world around us and the illnesses that affect us, while being closed to self-knowledge. We can be **resistant** to acknowledging our own personal reality, to taking up the challenge of change or to admitting and abdicating the gains that the studied condition brings us. Therefore, it may take more than one practice and activity to identify and embrace our symptoms and discomforts, especially when old and deep issues are involved.

It also takes **time** to understand ourselves, because often what is perceived as a difficulty is still only the tip of the self-research *iceberg*. When looking more closely, we begin to glimpse other needs, traits of temperament, discomforts and opportunities, which are related to the condition studied. In order to broaden our understanding of the condition under treatment, for example, a disease, we propose that the concerned consciousness apply the following questionnaire:

1. In what ways does this disease limit me?

2. What is it pushing me to learn?

3. How is it facilitating and helping me?

4. What elements do I think have contributed to its manifestation?

5. Which facts (intraphysical events) and parafacts (multidimensional events) is it related to in this life?

6. Which facts and parafacts is it related to prior to this life?

7. What personal traits are related to this illness?

8. What personal thosenes are related to this illness?

9. What behavioral traits inherited from the nuclear family have contributed to its manifestation?

10. What genetic traits have contributed to its manifestation?

11. What interpersonal conflicts have contributed to its manifestation?

Some books and sources help to reflect on the **meaning** of symptoms and diseases by proposing hypotheses for a correlation between health and the conflicts and needs symbolized by the body and mind. Even though they are generalizations, they help to expand the problem and are available for consultation by the reader, such as the seven books listed below:

1. The Healing Power of Illness: understanding what your symptoms are telling you, by Thorwald Dethlefsen and Rüdiger Dahlke[173].

2. *Krankheit als Sprache der Seele: Be-Deutung und Chance der Krankheitsbilder* [Illness as the language of the soul], by Rüdiger Dahlke[174].

3. Disease as a Symbol: Psychosomatics - the messages behind your symptoms, by Rüdiger Dahlke[175].

4. *La medicina patas arriba: ¿Y si Hamer tuviera razón?* [Medicine Upside Down: What If Hamer Was Right?], by Giorgio Mambretti and Jean Séraphim[152].

5. What your aches and pains are telling you: cries of the body, messages from the soul, by Michael Odoul[176].

6. Heal your body: the mental causes for physical illness and the metaphysical way to overcome them, by Louise L. Hay[177].

7. *La metamedicina* [Metamedicine], by Claudia Rainville[178].

However, the person should not be limited to seeking only cognitive and rationalized approaches in order to accept their reality, since some part of these conflicts will still remain inaccessible to their **conscious awareness**. To work in this hard-to-reach space, the path is to adopt approaches that directly access the emotional brain[53], such as meditation, mindfulness, reiki, massage, tuina, shiatsu, family constellation, microphysiotherapy, EFT (*Emotional Freedom Techniques*), psychoenergetic touch, EMDR and psychotherapy aimed at reliving and redefining memories.

The importance of harmony between the cognitive brain and the emotional brain in therapy is explained by psychiatrist David Servan-Schreiber. In his book "The Instinct to Heal"[53], already mentioned in chapter 2 of this book, he describes seven alternative treatment approaches for stress, anxiety and depression, which do not use medication or psychoanalysis, do not have their mechanism of action well understood and have remained outside the medical and psychiatry mainstream. The author's hypothesis is that such approaches act directly on the **emotional brain,** releasing accumulated trauma and pain that the cognitive brain is incapable of reshaping only through objective, logical and rational dialogue.

III. Move

The third stage produces movement, reorganization, recycling and the **change** of symptoms, difficulties, discomforts, illnesses or thosenes. The change begins with the choice of new objectives and goals, in relation to the five perspectives: physical, bioenergetic, emotional, mental and parapsychic. They can be changes in routine, life habits, behaviors or thosenes. As an example, listed below are 20 healthy habits and useful routines, which can make up the motivated person's neogoals, arranged from different perspectives:

A. Physical:

1. healthy eating;

2. physical activity;

3. relaxation practices;

4. sleep hygiene.

B. Energetic:

5. assimilation and deassimilation of energies;

6. control of the vibrational state;

7. energetic showers;

8. megaeuphorization, produced from the maximum exaltation of one's energies, and generating an aura of health.

C. Psychosomatic:

9. balanced affective-sexual relationship;

10. healthy conviviality;

11. healthy leisure;

12. reconciliation with those we feel disaffection.

D. Mentalsomatic:

13. meditation free of dogma, exemplified by mindfulness;

14. mental hygiene;

15. personal mentalsomatic task, by daily dedication to productive intellectual activities;

16. posture of Cosmoethical Sceptical Optimism (CSO).

E. Parapsychic:

17. development of personal parapsychic signals;

18. lucid projectability;

19. offiex;

20. penta.

Changing behaviors, habits and thosenes requires motivation and persistence, as it is a long-term process, at the risk of relapse. Therefore, the previous steps of identifying and embracing are fundamental, acting as true foundations, which consolidate the understanding of the problem experienced and sustain the desire to change the consciousness. The greater the **understanding** of how we function, from the physical, energetic, emotional, mental capacity to the parapsychic capacity, the better the results to incorporate changes will be. "The biggest and worst prisons are bad habits"[1:541][Translation].

Motivation for change can be organized into five levels, from pre-contemplation, when there is no intention to change; contemplation, in which it begins to be considered, but without a prediction of when it will actually begin; preparation, with the decision and plan to begin it within a month; action, when change is actively occurring; to maintenance, in which its consolidation takes place[179]. This model was initially developed in the 70s to assist people with addictions, but is currently applied to various behavioral changes, focusing on strategies to overcome the challenges characteristic of each level.

In addressing specific changes for a stage of life, geriatrician Dennis McCullough improved people's knowledge about the needs related to the last years of life and how to care for the **elderly**, integrating the family, caregivers, professionals and health resources. In the book My Mother, Your Mother[180], the author presents the eight seasons of late life and proposes ways to deal with them, based on his own experience in caring for his mother. The eight seasons are stability, commitment, crisis, recovery, decline, announcement of death, death and grief/legacy.

This need was recently discussed in an article published by Dr. Carla Rosane Ouriques Couto[r], in which she presents the journey

---

r   https://www.slowmedicine.com.br/delirium-sobre-as-nossas-maes/

she experienced with her hospitalized mother. During her hospital stay, she says that she needed to review her **attitude** as a daughter, woman, and physician so that her mother would receive proper care to treat a urinary tract infection, rather than the misdiagnosis of a psychiatric problem resulting from "careless medicine."

In the vicinity of death, recognizing the five phases of **grief** described by researcher Elizabeth Kubler-Ross (1926–2004) can also help to keep track of the feelings experienced due to the loss of a loved one. The phases characterized by denial, anger, bargaining, depression and acceptance are not linear, and can occur in different sequences and even with the absence of one or more phases. Some researchers already include other phases, or propose other models to understand grief. But, regardless of the framework adopted, the proposal here is to include grief and death as aspects to be discussed with yourself, family members and caregivers.

To optimize and maintain one's focus on change, guidance from experienced professionals is a valuable **resource**, for example, with support from psychotherapy, coaching, biofeedback, Cultivating Emotional Balance (CEB), Neurolinguistic Programming (NLP), among other practices. After all, as the American poet Robert Frost wrote, "...the best way out is always through".

Experimentation with techniques, practices and resources proposed by conscientiology also helps in the phase of change to reach a new level of self-care. Here, for example, are 60 conscientiological techniques, practices and tools, described in several publications indicated in this book, and suggested for study and application by the interested consciousness:

1. 1 more year of intraphysical life technique.

2. 10 basic personal values technique[121].

3. 10-day isolation technique.

4. 50 times more technique.

5. Admiration-disagreement binomial.

6. Antelucan work technique.

7. Basic Mobilization of Energies technique (BME).

8. Break of routine technique.

9. Breaking of conditionings technique[121].

10. Claritaskal irreverence technique.

11. Closed circulation of energies technique.

12. Consciential encapsulation.

13. Conscientiogram.

14. Conscientiological authorship.

15. Conscientiological teaching.

16. Conscientiological volunteering.

17. Conscientiotherapy.

18. Coronofrontochakral circuit technique.

19. Cosmogram technique.

20. Craniochakral voltaic arc technique.

21. Deintruding smile technique.

22. Duo's Code of Cosmoethics (DCC).

23. Eliminating unnecessary self-mimicry technique.

24. Energetic shower technique.

25. Parapsychic signals.

26. Evolutionary counterblow.

27. Evolutionary insinuations.

28. Examining one's contributions method.

29. Exhaustiveness technique.

30. Existential balance.

31. Existential inversion technique (invexis).

32. Existential recycling technique (recexis).

33. Five-hour self-reflection technique.

34. Group Code of Cosmoethics (GCC).

35. Guinea-pig conscin technique.

36. Homeostatic reference pattern technique.

37. Intention qualification technique.

38. Interassistantial self-pacification technique.

39. Invisible Colleges of conscientiology.

40. Law of greatest effort technique.

41. Lung expansion technique.

42. Megaeuphorization.

43. Offiex.

44. Parapsychic dynamics.

45. Parasurgery.

46. Penta.

47. Personal Code of Cosmoethics (PCC).

48. Personal Code of Generosity.

49. Prophylactic "it is not yet" technique.

50. Retrocognition.

51. Self-inventariogram technique.

52. Self-research laboratories.

53. Self-thosenation diary.

54. Shielded intraphysical base technique.

55. Sympathetic energetic deassimilation technique (sym-deas).

56. Tabula rasa technique.

57. Technique of forgiveness.

58. Techniques for lucid projetability.

59. Vibrational State (VS).

60. Waking physical immobility technique.

The set of therapeutic actions developed by the consciousness to achieve their desired goals, based on the FEMA method, make up the personalized **self-protocol.** The more detailed and structured this self-protocol is, the better it will reflect the specific reality of the person, optimizing their intimate recycling. Thus, the self-protocol is opposed to pre-structured protocols and individualizes care. At the same time, it is open to constant review and adjusted to the new experienced set of realities and contexts.

An interpretation of the results gained from the self-protocol can challenge traditional logic, due to **paradoxical responses** that occur when health is approached from other paradigms. Below, we cite six paradoxical responses, which demonstrate that the person, despite their apparent setback, may be advancing in their self-care:

1. **Worsening.** The aggravation or worsening of a person's health that, after explaining their conflicts and personal needs, deepens their self-knowledge, recovers their self-connection and promotes the recovery of their health.

2. **Slowness.** The slow improvement of an illness that naturally has a long recovery cycle, despite personal efforts to speed up this process. The frustrated expectation of a rapid improvement often hides the small achievements made towards healing.

3. **Reappearance.** The reappearance of an illness that the person has had in the past, during the treatment of a current condition, which suggests that both situations may be related. Different diseases can represent gradations of the same personal conflict, manifesting in a serial manner. In order to resolve it, the body will follow the opposite path, and may express symptoms that the person has not felt for many years.

4. **Chronicity.** The continuation of the chronic disease, despite the person's efforts to overcome it and eliminate the use of medicines and other associated care. Since chronic disease acts as a stabilizing factor of ongoing intimate recycling, it is not always possible to eliminate it without harming the recycling that is being carried out. In this case, the person allows themselves to live with the disease, based on their legitimate interest in overcoming the condition or personal conflict that triggered it.

5. **Balance.** The appearance of a new illness in the convalescent person that is required in order to rebalance the effects of the previous illness. For example, an acute intestinal infection arising in the final stage of recovery from a muscle injury. In this context, just as a disease can be the trigger for an evolutionary crisis, it can also be a resource for restoring better health at the end of the recently overcome disease.

6. **Terminal.** In terminal diseases, it is not possible for the person to recover their full health due to the natural deterioration

of the body, but other components of personal well-being that are being monitored and measured may be improving, such as providing comfort, self-love, understanding the meaning of the illness and the meaning of life, and the personal and familial preparation for the biological death of the consciousness.

IV. Again

The last step means to **start over**, restart or simply to go "again", and symbolizes the transition between the end of the current cycle and the beginning of the new cycle. The objective of dedicating a step to the transition of cycles is to demonstrate how self-care is dynamic and continuous, meeting the same principles of consciential health, and being in constant need of adaptation and flexibility by the consciousness, i.e., to find, embrace, move, then start all over again.

The presence of **willingness** at the end of each cycle can be expressed by the famous character Baby, from the iconic 90's American television series Dinosaurs, where the consciousness wishes *over and over and over again* to experience a new cycle with joy and enthusiasm. The mental attitude of this phase is also described by the "beginner's mind", valued in meditation and mindfulness practices, which enables us to look with curiosity at all situations, even though they are already apparently known to the individual.

The perspective of a fresh start implies an **attitude** of not rushing or skipping steps, because at the end of the cycle, a new one begins. The consciousness, therefore, does not "get rid" of the problem at the end of each cycle, but starts a new one. The best approach is then to value each step, even if they may overlap, as it is essential that it be carried out and conducted well to establish a new level of consciential health. The process is not simple and demands time, courage and attention from those who decide to expand their self-care and self-research possibilities.

In this sense, the self-care cycles resemble the ouroboros, represented by a serpent that eats its own tail, and which symbolizes the cycle of evolution, renewal and eternity. It is also similar to the premises of the **circularity** technique, proposed by Vieira[181], in which the consciousness uses multiple approaches to better understand the topic under study, and to apply it in favor of their own evolution:

> "The *circularity technique* is the use of didactic conscientiological research, through approaching the same complex subject in a multifaceted, cyclical manner, by dissecting, anatomizing and enriching with exhaustive enumerations and detail, little by little, the complexity of the structure regarding the content formed construct of the fact or phenomenon, parafact or paraphenomenon, in order to understand it better, organizing, in the end, the encyclopedic combination of various interactive evolutionary instruments, at the same time, in different areas of manifestation, specialties of conscientiology and qualities of megafocal themes"[181][Translation].

The theme of the new cycle may be from the same thematic axis, a variant of the previous theme, or it may even be a completely new theme. The arrangement of themes in the cycles can be represented by a basket full of **balls** of wool. Each ball represents a self-care theme and, for each cycle, the consciousness draws from the basket a ball, unrolls it as far as it can go, and reorganizes it. In the next cycle, they can take out the same ball of wool, continue the theme from the previous cycle, or get a completely new ball, and develop other personal aspects.

However, for each cycle, the consciousness does not resume from where they left off, but from a point higher on the scale of lucidity regarding their self-care, being more prepared and competent to support themselves and other evolutionary colleagues in this incessant **movement**. Such learning will be integrated into the consciousness' evolutionary intelligence, through which it understands and adapts better to human life[182].

In order to facilitate the organized planning and achieved results, these authors developed the Self-Care Canvas (Figure 3), which seeks to group the key points of each phase of the cycle into a single framework. The proposed Canvas can be customized, or it can be replaced by another **tool** that allows for the monitoring of self-care, according to each person's style and expertise. And it can also be used in conjunction with other support tools, such as recording information in a personal diary, filling out a daily checklist of tasks, maintaining one's health history on a timeline and adopting coping cards, among many others.

When recovering the case of pain presented in chapter 7, we filled out the Self-Care Canvas (Figure 4) based on a common situation, in order to facilitate the understanding of how to use this tool. In this case, the person experiences a headache that bothers them, recognizes the possibility of including new care practices and understands the influence of their life routine on the way their pain is expressed. The questions promote reflection and help the person to develop answers that guide them in **applying** the FEMA method.

Figure 3. Self-Care Canvas.

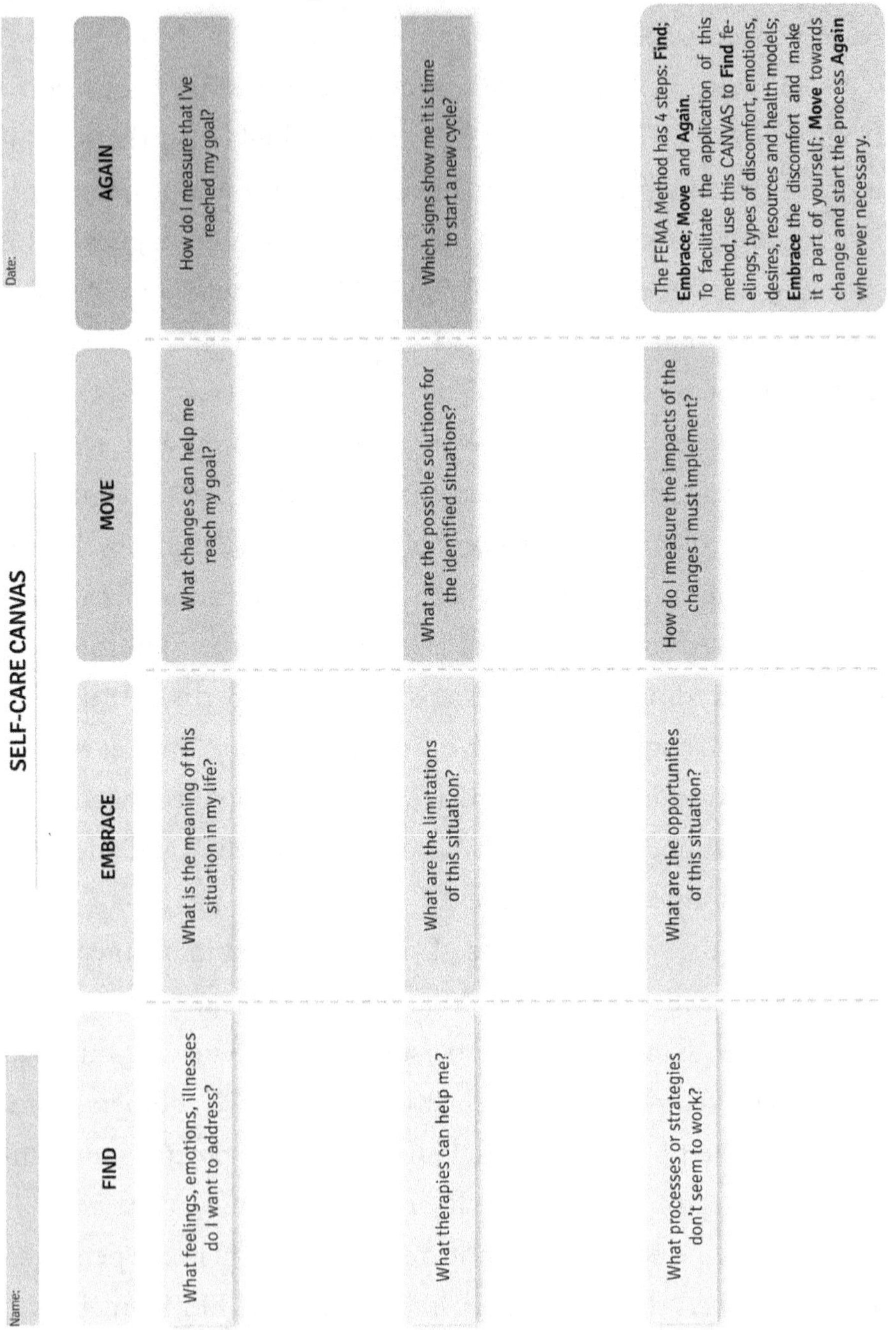

SELF-CARE CANVAS

Name:

Date:

FIND	EMBRACE	MOVE	AGAIN
What feelings, emotions, illnesses do I want to address?	What is the meaning of this situation in my life?	What changes can help me reach my goal?	How do I measure that I've reached my goal?
What therapies can help me?	What are the limitations of this situation?	What are the possible solutions for the identified situations?	Which signs show me it is time to start a new cycle?
What processes or strategies don't seem to work?	What are the opportunities of this situation?	How do I measure the impacts of the changes I must implement?	

The FEMA Method has 4 steps: **Find**; **Embrace**; **Move** and **Again**.
To facilitate the application of this method, use this CANVAS to **Find** feelings, types of discomfort, emotions, desires, resources and health models; **Embrace** the discomfort and make it a part of yourself; **Move** towards change and start the process **Again** whenever necessary.

Download at www.autocuidado.org/blog

Figure 4. An example of a completed Self-Care Canvas.

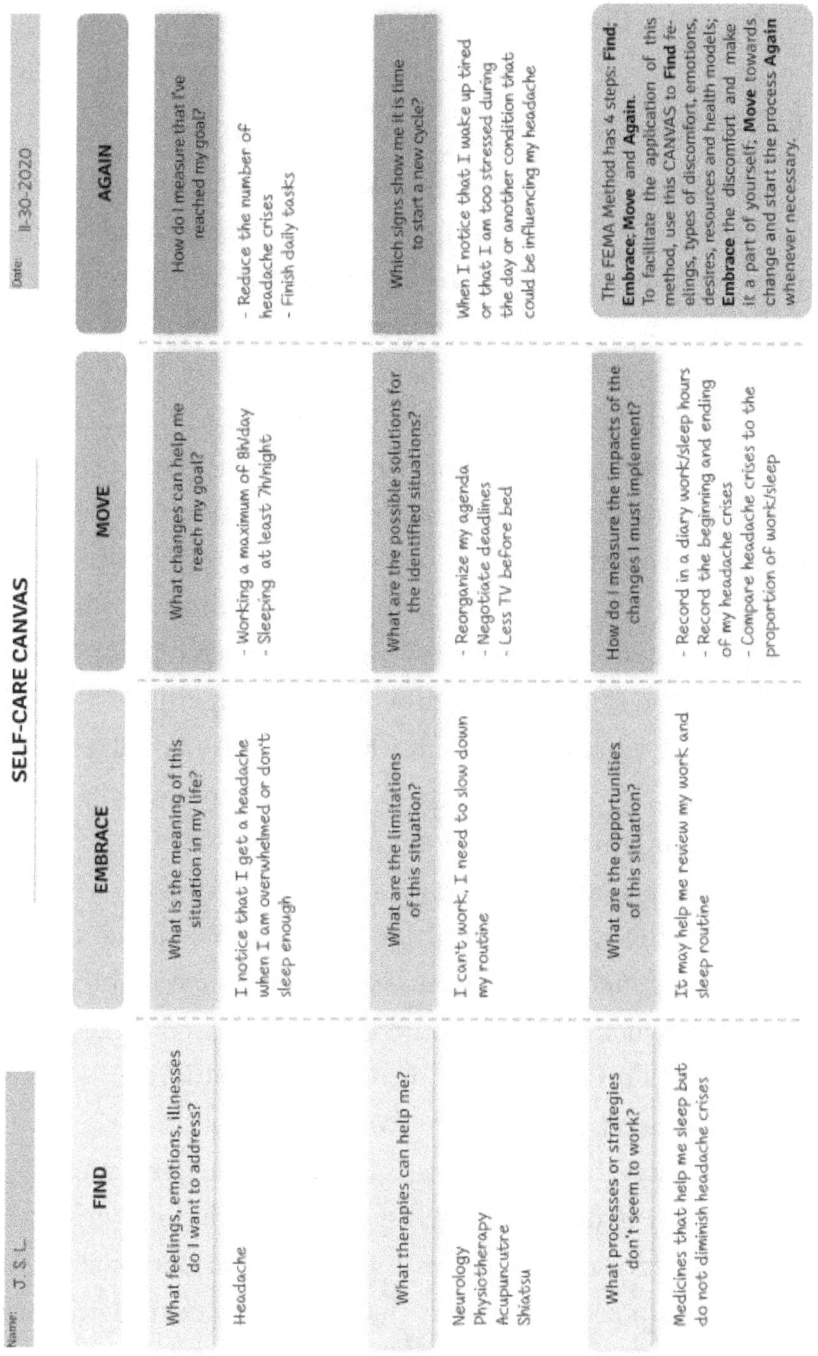

The **application** of the FEMA method in practice is demonstrated in the health history of Anastasius.

The Case of Anastasius

Anastasius has always been a dedicated sportsman. He trained many hours a week, participated in competitions, but repeatedly had muscle injuries during training that required him to reduce his pace and prevented him from competing. He sought conventional treatment, with orthopedics and physiotherapy, but the injuries continued, although no reason was found to justify the injuries. The lack of answers and results led him to look for other ways of addressing the problem, when seeking out a holistic therapist. In therapy, he found other possible interpretations for the health problem he was experiencing when reflecting on the meaning of his illness. What was his body telling him? What conflict was represented in his symptoms? What personal need was he not attending? The search to understand what the problem was, what was needed to improve himself, which professionals could support him and what was the meaning behind his illness represents the *Find* step.

In therapy, he realized that, while sport occupied a large part of his life, living with his family and other professional challenges were not being met. From this understanding, he was able to notice the benefits that the disease could bring him by connecting better with himself. This moment of introjecting the disease and making it a part of you, characterizes the *Embrace* stage.

From there, he made changes in his routine to balance his dedication to these issues. He started spending more time with his family, dedicated himself to a professional project and looked for other ways of harmonizing the anxiety that previously overflowed into his sport. These initiated actions mark the *Move* step.

A few months later, he started experiencing another muscle injury that was even more limiting and painful than the previous one. At that moment, Anastasius was confused, was he doing *everything wrong*? If he was on the right track, why was he getting worse? The need to restart a new self-care cycle characterized the *Again* step.

He then sought help again to interpret what he was going through and, when assessing the possible meaning of these new symptoms, he realized that they were related to some inability in dealing with family and professional situations that had been triggered from the moment he began to devote more time to these two axes in his life. The move to seek answers and support defines a new step, *Find*.

That's when he realized that the new illness was a part of him, and a result of the move he was making to meet the needs he had learned about during the previous illness. The disease had evolved because he had also advanced in his ability to meet his needs. If before, he had avoided noticing them, now he had difficulties in conducting initiatives with balance and was able to perceive his anxiety at work. Such understanding dispelled his anxieties and brought him new encouragement to continue pursuing his self-care. He also used his references to make new adjustments, in his familial and professional performance. To further broaden his understanding of health, he began reading the book: What Your Aches and Pains Are Telling You, by Michael Odoul[176]. Appropriating the disease to the changes one is making in one's life brings a feeling of belonging and motivation that drives one's personal mobilization, marking a new stage, *Embrace*.

Understanding the points that still needed to be refined allowed him to draw up a new strategy of action, which involved treatment of the disease itself, and a new adjustment to how he interacted with his family and his ongoing professional projects. The recovery process was not linear, and there were times when he went overboard with his physical rehabilitation, and the pain got worse. But these fluctuations served as triggers for further adjustments in treatment. The initiatives and adjustments in treatment signal a new phase, *Move*.

Gradually, the pain was decreasing and, when he was almost released for light training, he experienced a severe intestinal infection, accompanied by diarrhea, which limited him and caused him to lose more than 6 pounds. To treat this new disease, he sought medical help, which helped him to recover. The appearance of this new crisis in one's personal health marks the *Again* step.

But, contrary to what happened in the other health crises, this time, Anastasius was not perplexed about feeling sick. The illness naturally made sense to him, as it felt like a great cleansing to purify him of all the accumulated pain, tension, and even weight, which he had gained during the treatment period. To check his understanding of what this disease would represent in terms of his personal history, he sought information in books and on the internet, which helped him confirm his way of thinking. This time, Anastasius conducted the *Find* and *Embrace* steps, without needing a professional to help him decode the meaning of what he was experiencing.

When commenting with his wife that this disease had been good for him, she found it strange, but her disbelief did not shake his conviction: the illness had its purpose. Recovered from the infection, he felt well and was ready to restart his training sessions, and to reconcile practicing sport with the other aspects of his life.

The steps of the FEMA method can be didactically **organized** by the 5W2H tool, according to the following table:

Table 5. FEMA method organized by the 5W2H tool.

Step	Find	Embrace	Move	Again
What?	**Find** Identify Search Look for	**Embrace** Recognize Realize	**Move** Change Transform Recycle	**Again** Restart "begin again"
Why?	Recognizing that there is a discomfort* and identifying what it is allows you to act and transform it.	Embracing discomfort makes it a part of you, and empowers you to change it by changing yourself.	Transforming discomfort requires breaking through inertia, moving towards change.	Self-care has no end.
Where?	At home, at work, on the road, in self-research laboratories, in therapeutic care, in the extraphysical dimension and wherever the consciousness manifests themselves.			
When?	When noticing unidentified discomfort.	When feeling strange about the discomfort, and wishing to avoid it, deny it, or treat it as unworthy.	When identifying desired goals and targets in relation to the discomfort experienced.	When completing a cycle.
Who?	By the consciousness themself, with the support of family members, friends, therapists, extraphysical helpers and other consciousnesses predisposed to assistance.			
How?	Self-research based on an integrative and consciential approach, considering three factors: genetics, paragenetics, mesology; and five perspectives: physical, bioenergetic, emotional, mental and parapsychic. With the application of different medical rationales, complementary therapies, techniques and resources of self-research. With specialized therapeutic support, according to the interest and need.			
How much?	Attributes: self-effort and dedication. Time: hours of self-research. Energy: psychic and consciential. Money: varies according to the choice of resources, practices and therapies.			

*Discomfort, in this table, represents any changes, symptoms, difficulties, discontent, anxieties, diseases, illnesses, imbalances, weaktraits, absentraits, or thosenes that demand attention; and interests, desires, strongtraits, insights and inspirations.

In order to expand the **possibilities** of self-care practices and self-research stimuli, besides consulting the content described in this book, it is important to remain neophilic. The development of consciential health is dynamic, and new practices and techniques are presented and researched daily, including by you. This is our invitation: to develop your own self-care practices, experiment, disseminate, publish and contribute to the *corpus* of integrative health.

Do you identify any opportunities for *expanding* your self-care practices? What *tools* do you already use for this? How can you *apply* the **FEMA method** to yourself and others in *developing self-care*?

Chapter 9
Self-awareness and Self-research

In your daily life, are you invited to *think about yourself*? How do you approach this? How do you develop your *self-research*? The objectives of this chapter are to present self-research as a *tool* for **self-knowledge** and **self-care**, and to encourage the reader to develop **self-awareness** and experience daily life by applying more *lucidity and scientificity*.

Since antiquity, the approach to self-awareness has generated concerns and confrontation. The couplet ***"know thyself"*** (from the original Greek, *gnōthi seauton*), inscribed at the entrance of the temple of Apollo, already encouraged this way of thinking in visitors from the ancient world, who went in search of the prophecies of the Pythias of the famous Oracle of Delphi, in Ancient Greece.

In this same temple, Socrates would have been declared the wisest man, giving rise to the popular Socratic paradox *"I only know that I know nothing"*, which many scholars claim was never said by him. Nevertheless, this phrase sums up one of the Socratic premises: that the recognition of one's **ignorance** is essential for obtaining knowledge.

The resulting process of knowing and understanding oneself is called **self-knowledge,** and encompasses one's personal paradigm, temperament, behavior, motivations and interests, thosenity, strongtraits-weaktraits-absentraits, and, expanded beyond this life, one's holobiography and personal holomemory. It is closely related to the development of self-awareness, as an agent of this capacity to perceive and know oneself.

Self-awareness was presented by Kant[s] as awareness of the self as an agent of thought and knowledge of reality and, according to Hegel[t], as the awareness that the self acquires of itself when it recognizes itself as an agent of external reality, seen in conformity with its own reflection. According to Vieira:

> "Self-awareness is the faculty or capacity whereby the human being is aware of his/her existence, or is aware of being conscious of his/her mind, thoughts and sentiments. This involves other mental faculties such as reason, memory and imagination." [67:238].

Self-knowledge and self-awareness have different **meanings**, and are usually differentiated by the first referring to knowledge itself and the second indicating the consciousness in relation to itself, which facilitates the construction of this knowledge. For some researchers, they may be adopted as synonyms and, in popular usage,

---

s   https://plato.stanford.edu/entries/kant/
t   https://plato.stanford.edu/entries/hegel/

it is not uncommon for them to be treated with the same meaning. They also coexist with other concepts of a similar meaning, such as self-cognition and self-diagnosis. They also interact with mental functions or faculties, such as attention, memory, lucidity and discernment, with practical relations of proximity between the concepts.

Although the two words have concrete differences, in practice they interact continuously, and it is difficult to characterize their differences during the experience of a person's own investigation. Discerning between self-knowledge and the awareness of oneself that provides this knowledge is, to some extent, a theoretical **distinction**, as the knowledge produced is incorporated into one's self-awareness that provides new knowledge.

However, the refinement in distinguishing these concepts allows the person to discriminate between the ability to observe themselves and the content observed. The exercise of being aware of one's behavior and understanding it provides a deeper understanding of **self-research**. As a result, it drives recins (intraconsciential recycling), toward the goals desired by the consciousness, whether related to self-qualification, self-realization, or to improving one's health and personal care. "Self-conscientiality balances one's life"[1:151][Translation].

Through self-research, each person can build answers to personal questions, reducing the *guesswork* and moving closer to a most accurate analysis of themselves. Such discoveries represent the most advanced or leading-edge **relative truths** regarding the consciousness' current moment, resulting from their personal capacity to understand their reality, in the process of increasing self-knowledge and self-awareness.

On the path of self-awareness, we admit human **similarities**, while recognizing the uniqueness of each consciousness, and the limitations of Western science in providing such interconnected knowledge into the intangible and multifaceted universe of our personality.

Science is better at recognizing human patterns than at explaining exceptions. In this context, self-research also allows one to study personal **singularities**, still little studied by science, as being exceptions, outgrowths or extrapolations in the daily manifestations of consciousnesses on this planet.

In this way, self-research transforms the view of people and the world around us, expanding our **cosmovision**. Knowing yourself favors the understanding of the other, but the effects do not stop there. Self-acceptance favors accepting the other, and self-qualification enhances your personal ability to help qualify other people.

Self-research is the study or research of one's own consciousness, by oneself, employing all available research instruments, at the same time, in the consciousness' intimacy and in the cosmos[75:81]. It aims to develop self-knowledge and self-awareness in order to achieve personal evolutionary goals[183].

By exhaustively and continuously researching themself in a personal and participative way, the consciousness promotes a correction of its self-image, the anatomization of intimate conflicts and pedagogical **self-restructuring**, based on self-teaching and personal re-education. The achieved personal recycling also impacts people around the researcher, and can serve as inspiration and motivation to follow the path of self-research, towards self-development.

In this way, the consciousness experiences an increase in altruism, combats childish self-centeredness and gradually improves their personal **self-criticism,** while acquiring *self-distrust* or *critical judgment*[184].

Building self-knowledge requires that people research themselves from a paradigm and method compatible with their **object** of study: the consciousness itself. In self-research, scientific knowledge is the starting point to broaden *knowledge about oneself*, based on the understanding of leading-edge relative truths (verpons). However, proof of the formulated theories is only carried out with self-experimentation[183].

At this moment, there is an **inversion** of logic in producing verpons, when the truth starts to be developed in the person, within their experiences, to the detriment of knowledge that is outside them[185:902]. Carl Rogers[146:23] synthesizes this supremacy by stating that *"Experience is, for me, the highest authority"*. Such self-experimentation transforms and supports the personal neoparadigm of the consciousness[1:59].

Here are three **differentiators** of self-research compared to biomedical science epistemology:

1. The consciousness dedicates themselves to the subject-matter that it wishes, gradually **freeing** themselves from the prevailing preferences and directions of science-media-religion.

2. The consciousness achieves **autonomy** in constructing their own knowledge, without relying on heteroresearch and knowledge produced by others.

3. The consciousness goes deep into their own very personal **essence** that is unique in the Cosmos, and finds answers that only apply to themselves.

The process of self-research is structured in different formats and **steps**, which resemble other research methods, and can be organized into the five steps described by researcher Adriana Kauati[183] and exemplified by researchers Patrícia Gaion[186] and Hernande Leite[112]:

1. **Problem definition:** identify the objective and problem you want to solve.

2. **Literature review:** search for literature papers in order to facilitate the association of ideas and the elaboration of verpons.

3. **Data collection:** register and gather records, in the form of annotations, typed and personal notes made during readings, which make up the Self-researcher's Notebook[184], to which you can apply questionnaires, tests, comparisons, interviews and inventories, like the examples of the tools listed in chapter 8.

4. **Experiment:** plan and apply experiments to deepen the research, verify hypotheses, or overcome the identified problem, with the support of techniques, laboratories and other resources that already exist or are developed from the researcher's creativity.

5. **Analysis of results:** throughout the research, analyze the findings of the review, collection and experimentation stages, formulate self-diagnostic hypotheses to be verified, characterize the limitations of the research and synthesize its conclusions.

Self-research starts with a **question** that points to gaps in self-knowledge, which becomes the problem to be investigated. These personal questions *say a lot* about you, your interests and your desires. They are a measurement unit of self-awareness, capable of indicating the balance of your existence[1:417]. In the FEMA method, they make up the first step: Find.

The **self-willingness** to find the answers demands living with doubts and uncertainties, and has roots in personal ignorance. It also requires courage to *dive deep* inside yourself, increasing your *stamina* with the practice of reflection and introspection. It should also include embracement as a way to understand the characteristics and singularities of the individual, exercised in the second stage of the FEMA method: Embrace.

Experimentation occurs in a programmed manner, but also in a spontaneous and unexpected way, made possible by the contingencies and synchronicities of everyday life. The lucidity to identify and the openness to take advantage of these experiences speeds up the research and brings insights regarding new experiments. Promoting change and seeking solutions is part of the process of moving and starting again whenever necessary, present in steps 3 and 4 of the FEMA method: Move and Again.

Research findings are more reliable when **recorded**, without requiring the memory to retain the details of the events. The researcher writes down the relevant facts, including what they do not yet understand, with an interest to understanding them in the future. At first, it is more difficult to know which ideas, insights and experiences are important to the ongoing research, and it is worth the effort to register *more than less*. Ideas that are overlooked will not have a chance to be analyzed[1:401]. The optimization of records occurs with the practice and adoption of personal techniques, such as these seven:

1. The adoption of personal **codes** in recording facts.

2. Keep a pen and paper always within **reach** of your hand, pocket or bag.

3. Keep **notebooks** in fixed places in the house, such as on your office desk and at your bedside.

4. The practice of taking notes in **thematic diaries**, focused on interests under research, such as diaries on reflections, food, health, menstruation, projective experiences, a dream diary, etc.

5. The use of **mobile** apps that enable voice recording, file typing, or freehand writing.

6. With very long experiences, start recording with **keywords** or milestones of the experience and then fill the report with details.

7. The **standardization** of records, containing day, time, location and other references, positioned in the same sequence.

An **analysis** of the findings requires boldness to distance yourself from your *comfort zone* and face yourself. We must allow ourselves to discard hypotheses, deconstruct assumptions and refute obsolete truths. At this time, relying on the support of friends, health professionals, therapists, caregivers and other researchers to dialogue and debate broadens your evaluation perspectives and reduces your risk of *self-deception*.

The **conclusions** reached in the self-research allow you to update your own *instruction manual* and is an opportunity for personal renewal and *upgrading* to a new version, with the 2.0, 3.0 model, and so on, within your personal holobiography.

The **synergy** generated by self-effort in your self-research and overcoming growth crises leads to the refinement of personal skills in performing science for yourself and for others and to the maturing of research. Such skills help the self-researcher to qualify their self-perception to build increasingly reliable knowledge, in resonance with self-scientificity.

Self-scientificity is the quality of scientificity applied in self-research, by conducting an investigation of oneself, in an experiential and systematic way, based on the researcher's own conception of what science is. The scientific framework, when verified, increases the accuracy of the discoveries and allows the self-researcher to first examine the events, and then extract useful conclusions from the facts, eliminating the influence of beliefs or dogmas.

However, characterizing what **science** is, its attributes, methods and instruments, is challenging, as it is constantly changing. In addition to all the development of knowledge characterized in previous chapters, contemporary criteria transform classical scientific conceptions of how to produce it, for example, by proposing a progressive research program, methodological pluralism, or the fusion of natural and social areas[187]. At the same time, these criteria provoke new perspectives on self-awareness and self-research.

Therefore, there is no single scientific **model** to be followed, whether in research or self-research. It will be up to the researcher to choose the elements that are most compatible with their temperament and the subject under investigation, when experiencing personal scientificity.

Self-scientificity also denotes the coordinated application of intelligence, skills and personal attributes during self-research. Your *personal performance* shows which of these traits are most relevant to yourself, while also specifying self-development opportunities capable of driving self-research. To support the personal analysis, it is possible to indicate at least 15 qualifying **attributes** of self-scientificity, listed below[188]:

1. Antidogmatism.
2. Autodidactism.
3. Bibliophilia.
4. Disbelief.

5. Intellectuality.

6. Logic.

7. Neophilia.

8. Omniquestioning.

9. Openness.

10. Parapsychism.

11. Rationality.

12. Scientificity.

13. Self-criticism.

14. Self-discernment.

15. Technicality.

By acting more efficiently in understanding their personal attributes, the consciousness expands the *gauge* of thosenes and personal cognition, as well as the limit of applied self-scientificity. In practice, most **obstacles**, brakes and bottlenecks in self-research are related to the researcher's limitations and not to the structure of the research. "*There are self-ignored weaktraits*"[1:406][Translation].

Among the common obstacles are pride and personal **whims**, when the researcher avoids what is priority in their research to maintain some secondary benefit. Although they are already able to glimpse more promising paths, they are not willing to pay the expected toll. The price may be prestige, social standing, peer recognition, financial gain, or more intimate aspects, such as giving up dysfunctional relationships, behaviors, preferences, predilections or personal manias[1:482].

Another obstacle is the personal **blind spot,** which occurs when the researcher is not able to see how a personal trait is expressed, despite living with its effects on themselves and in social circles. The aspect that is unrecognized by self-observation generates confusion, because the person is not able to understand the unsatisfactory results experienced, and often imposes on others the responsibility for the failures it triggers from the, as yet unknown, expressed trait.

But how to search for what you don't see? An alternative is to act like astronomers, who, upon finding **anomalies** in the orbits of the planets, suspect that there is a celestial body that interferes in that natural and expected trajectory. Although this body cannot be seen, it is possible to define its characteristics (such as mass, gravitational field, etc.) by the distortion generated in the orbit under study.

In practice, consciential blind spots are expressed by **dissonances** or inconsistencies between their intention, the self-efforts applied and the results achieved. *The difference between the path traced and the location reached* can denote unconscious interference generated by personal traits that are in your blind spot.

Other people's reactions, impacts and responses to our actions are *feedback* concerning our intentions and traits. Performing a conjunctural analysis on the coherence of these findings exercises our cosmovision, by considering how the interaction of apparently isolated aspects contribute to a wider comprehension regarding our personal manifestation. *"Effects dissect intentions"*[1:414][Translation].

Advancing our understanding of blind spots will also require recycling ego defense mechanisms and other **adaptive mechanisms** that conceal our true interests and motivations. They represent solutions built by the person themselves, which bring comfort and security, but which trap them in working models that are incompatible with their real goals. Despite having been useful in the past, such behaviors are already starting to hinder more than help in self-development. Letting go of these mechanisms requires letting go of personal beliefs and traits from where they are anchored. However, in order to overcome these mechanisms, it is worth being cautious of the first answers that come to our mind about our motivations, intentions, interests and ways of acting, as they tend to still be distorted and impregnated by such mechanisms.

The renewal of our paradigm and personal belief system, through evolutionary libertarian self-research, prevents the paradoxical conditions of the neophobic scientist, the religious or mystical scientist, the superstitious scientist and the idolatrous self-scientist[188]. To this end, self-scientificity demands deconstructing at least five fallacies or **myths** of science:

1. Myth of **independence.** No research is carried out with complete independence, due to interactions with people, ideas, scientific findings and energies. Self-sufficiency is not independence, but interdependence led by the consciousness.

2. Myth of **limitation.** The limit of science is not imposed by the paradigm or method, but by the consciousness that has been restricted to the adopted paradigm and method. Ultimately, there is no science with limitations, but researchers who impose their limitations on the science they practice.

3. Myth of **neutrality.** There is no neutral science, because, despite the researcher's efforts not to interfere and act impartially, they influence the research results, even in an unsconscius way.

4. Myth of **objectivity.** Science is impregnated with the subjectivity inherent in the researcher who develops critical thinking, choices, judgments, beliefs and experiences.

5. Myth of **theoretical research.** There is no completely the-

oretical research, because, even if it does not present practical actions during the investigation, it intervenes at least in the researcher's personal universe, transforming their perspective, worldview and interaction with reality.

Myths and beliefs are the result of a lack of experience with the Principle of Disbelief (PD), in self-research and in daily life. When employed, the PD prompts the consciousness to rebuild the **bases** on which their personal ideas and conceptions are constructed. By questioning and reviewing the paradigm itself, the ideas become unstable and those more closely related to the new model in formation are left remaining.

In the process of change, *gaps* between the neoideas and the more entrenched retroparadigms of the consciousness will occur, triggering intimate conflicts until the **neoparadigm** is re-positioned and assumed. The difficulty of assuming a new model that is better and more optimized to the reality of the consciousness, seems to be a paradoxical answer, but it finds reasons in the intimate structure of the consciousness. The paradigm conflict syndrome[189], characterized by a personal crisis in abdicating an obsolete reference of yourself and experiencing the consciential paradigm, helps in the study of this condition.

An instrument used in self-research for the renovation of one's personal model is the Self-paradigmatic **Transition** Diagram[190]. The diagram proposes a method to define, formulate or design the different self-paradigmatic benchmarks, prompting the consciousness to reflect on the effects of the references adopted now and, in the past, in addition to the benefits of accomplishing a new transition.

Observing reality through another paradigm radically transforms personal conflicts and suffering, and can direct and even promote them to evolutionary assets or drivers. An example is when the person feels like a *fish out of water*, and doesn't feel as if they belong to their birth context or identify with the values of the society in which they are inserted. If, in this condition, such a person admits multidimensionality, they may support the hypothesis that this feeling of inadequacy and consciential *banishment* is due to a longing for their community of extraphysical origin, their *para*origin, which is more advanced in terms of values and interests. The perception of estrangement from the social context in which they are inserted takes on another meaning and represents a real condition of foreignness. From then on, the consciousness suffers less, by admitting a concrete reason that explains the myriad of conflicting feelings that characterize the **foreigner syndrome** in practice[191].

The paradigm guides the consciousness' gaze towards reality, as if looking through a **kaleidoscope.** *Just by rotating it the image changes.* This condition reinforces the popular saying: *everything is a matter of perspective.* Therefore, it is worth embracing a new paradigm that broadens one's self-understanding and promotes self-care and self-healing, through self-research and the experience of personal recycling.

Ultimately, this ability demonstrates the consciousness' level of evolutionary intelligence to distance themselves from the common "truths" of the intraphysical dimension, in search of **priority truths** regarding their own evolution, with positive effects in inter-assistance and consciential exemplarism.

Among the various types of intelligence already proposed, evolutionary intelligence characterizes the personal ability to understand how **evolution** occurs in the Cosmos, not only regarding the biological aspect, addressed by Darwinism, but also from the perspective of the consciousness.

Evolutionary intelligence is closely related to other types of intelligence already studied, especially intrapersonal, interpersonal and existential intelligence, but it cannot be used as a synonym for any of them. According to its proposer Waldo Vieira:

> "Evolutionary intelligence (EI) is the ability to apprehend, learn or understand and adapt to human life, based on the self-aware theorical application and expansion of the already assimilated consciential, personal mechanism of evolution, including cosmoethicology, seriexology and proexology, defining the consciousness' self-discernment regarding their rational consciential evolution, including lucid self-evolution, in the dynamization of their own self-thosenic and cosmoethical performance"[182][Translation].

Such intelligence is **key** for those who wish to live better in this human dimension, in line with the universal evolutionary laws that govern the consciousness' personal renewal, expression and interrelationships. After all, *those who embrace and understand the observed facts gain more*, even if contrary to their will, rather than dedicating their personal efforts to deny reality.

From the perspective of evolutionary intelligence, evolution is very long-term sequential work, in which it is not possible to *skip steps*. But that doesn't make it disagreeable. Moments of joy and pleasure in daily self-overcoming, in understanding reality itself, neo-overpons, the sharing of mutual learning and the feeling of belonging to interassistantial work are among the small revitalizing **evolutionary achievements** capable of, little by little, consolidating evolutionary shifts. The understanding of oneself and human life goes through at least three phases, forming a crescendo[1:508]:

1. **Submission.** The acceptance of knowledge subordinated to others, received through indoctrination, dogmatism and brainwashing.

2. **Autodidacticism.** Theoretical knowledge acquired by oneself, through reading and the self-taught consulting of audiovisual materials, even without field research.

3. **Self-research.** Erudition coming from one's personal research and lucid self-experience by exploring reality for oneself.

Self-research is inherent in human learning and evolution. It is born from the consciousness' intrinsic desire and necessity to develop knowledge for themselves of life around them. When considering the phases of understanding yourself and the scientific method, it can be considered that self-research is expressed by the **experience** of, for example, any of the following 12 occurrences, arranged in an increasing logical scale:

1. **Identification.** You identify ideas, facts and phenomena that are still misunderstood, but show no interest in understanding them.

2. **Interest.** Misunderstood facts draw your attention, and you show an interest in understanding them.

3. **Singularities.** You begin to increase your curiosity and express satisfaction when faced with anomalies, dissonances, paradoxes and singularities.

4. **Doubt.** You develop questions, but still doesn't see any answers.

5. **Relationships.** You develop relationships between the topic under study and other facts and perceptions.

6. **Analysis.** You make hypotheses for your questions, but don't conclude anything.

7. **Experimentation.** You test and prove hypotheses to support your analysis.

8. **Summary.** You define a hypothesis and understand the subject-matter in a timely manner.

9. **Interrelationships.** You build interrelationships between the topic under study and other research areas.

10. **Expansion.** You expand your understanding of the broader context regarding the topic under study, in dynamic interaction with other observed realities.

11. **Verpon.** You share your discoveries with your social network, with a genuine interest in listening to opposing and divergent points of view.

12. **Disbelief.** You review your analysis and adjust your conclusions based on new events and experiences.

In the evolutionary process, the consciousness first discards their beliefs and reviews their personal paradigm, to then recycle their **temperament**[1.447]. Such recycling, in general, requires effort and experiences accumulated over multiple lives to be consolidated. However, the benefits are felt from the very first steps of change.

Harmony and balance gradually grow in one's personal expression, with the polishing of one's temperament. The **progressive expression** of homeostatic traits reveals this evolution in daily life, for example, through the predominance of the first column, in the following 25 comparisons:

Table 6. Comparison of homeostatic and nosographic traits.

No	Balance/harmony	Imbalance/disharmony
1	Benignity	Malice
2	Coherence	Incoherence
3	Concessions	Demands
4	Constancy	Inconstancy
5	Cosmoethics	Anticosmoethics
6	Cosmovision	Monovison
7	Discernment	Madness
8	Flexibility	Rigidity
9	Fraternism	Selfishness
10	Freedom	Bondage
11	Generosity	Avarice
12	Good mood	Bad mood
13	Gratitude	Ingratitude
14	Healthy conviviality	Unhealthy conviviality
15	Imperturbability	Intimate conflict
16	Lucidity	Mental confusion
17	Neophilia	Neophobia
18	Openness	Closed-mindedness
19	Optimism	Pessimism
20	Organization	Disorganization
21	Prudence	Imprudence
22	Tranquility	Anxiety
23	Understanding	Misunderstanding
24	Universalism	Preconceptions
25	Wisdom	Ignorance

In this way, scientific research dedicated to understanding the functioning of the mind, brain and temperament is able to accelerate self-research and personal recycling. **Neuroscience** research focusing on the organization of thought, logical analysis, decision-making and cognitive biases, for example, works in the way of a brain and mind user manual. It reveals how we can better use our cognition and provides an understanding of how our brain works, breaking down myths and inviting us to take a fresh perspective. The published studies presented below demonstrate the importance of these findings:

1. The book **Thinking**, Fast and Slow, in which Daniel Kahneman[192] differentiates intuitive from deliberative thinking and explains the factors involved in how we build our conclusions and make decisions.

2. The article published by researchers Gunes Sevinc and Sara W. Lazar[193], which demonstrates how the application of **mindfulness** is capable of promoting ethical attitudes in those who practice it.

3. The book **Love** 2.0: Finding Happiness and Health in Moments of Connection, in which researcher Barbara L. Fredrickson[194] redefines what love is, as a momentary experience of connection between people that produces a shared positive emotion. It also reveals the interactions between love and body biochemistry, neuroplasticity, and mental faculties such as resilience and empathy. It deepens the importance of self-love and introduces practices to develop more moments of connection in everyday life.

4. Studies in **psychoneuroimmunology**, conducted by Andrea Marques-Deak and Esther Sternberg[195], which demonstrate the two-way communication paths between the neuroendocrine, neurological and immune systems.

5. The collection of books by social scientist Brené Brown that addresses the power of **vulnerability**: Daring Greatly[196], Rising Strong[197] and The Gifts of Imperfection[198], among others.

Self-research, strictly speaking, is **free**, non-partisan, independent from any type of religion, doctrine, scientific discipline or area of knowledge. However, different strands of human knowledge approach self-knowledge and self-researchaccording to their paradigms, principles and technologies. Next, the concepts for the theory and practice of self-research in the science of conscientiology are explored.

Conscientiological Self-research

According to conscientiology, birth in a new physical body **restricts the lucidity** of the consciousness, with a temporary loss of memories and knowledge already gained in previous physical and extraphysical experiences. If it were possible to mathematize this lucidity, each unit of knowledge would be represented by a *con*. For example, a lexical *con* represents the vocabulary units that the consciousness uses to communicate, and can be increased by learning a new language.

The loss and recovery of ***cons*** are natural effects of the rebirth cycles, so that not all self-knowledge achieved in this life is properly new. Much of the knowledge gained by self-research rescues memories and ideas that were forgotten when reborn. However, not every past *con* is useful in the current existence, within the assortment of data accumulated in the holomemory. The most advanced and priority *cons* originate from extraphysical experiences during the period of lucid intermission and, when recalled, ensure the achievement of the existential program[199].

In contrast, there are temporarily disabled, blocked and unrecoverable *cons* in this lifetime. These are the **anticons**, which remain encrypted and inaccessible for the protection of the consciousness. Among the examples of anticons are our past abuses, often against close family members, whose forgetfulness favors reconciliation.

In this process, conscientiological self-research predisposes, in addition to accessing cons and anticons, access to knowledge so far unexplored and unknown to the consciousness, or **neocons**. These *cons* demand neosynapses from the self-researcher, the greatest guinea pig of themselves, to understand the accessed neoverpons and to face their self-conflicts and self-corruptions that have been *brought to light*.

The mobilized recins, based on the genuine will and intention of self-overcoming, refine one's self-awareness regarding well-being and intimate harmony, that is, self-conscientiality. Thus, conscientiological self-research promotes the refinement of various types of **self-conscientiality,** such as the 16 proposed by Vieira[200], and listed below:

1. **Bioenergetic:** energosomatic; self-defending.
2. **Cosmoethical:** moral; incorrupt; upright.
3. **Deintruding:** therapeutic; discerning.
4. **Evolutionary:** recycling; inversive.
5. **Generic:** female; male.
6. **Graphic:** authorial; clarifying.
7. **Heuristic:** innovative; creative.
8. **Intellectual:** mentalsomatic.
9. **Interassistantial:** pentable.

10. **Mature:** adult; veteran; experienced; formed.

11. **Organizational:** disciplinarian.

12. **Parapsychic:** sensitive; multidimensional.

13. **Political:** sociological.

14. **Polykarmic:** egokarmic; groupkarmic; holokarmic.

15. **Somatic:** intraphysical; physiological.

16. **Verbal:** colloquial; idiomatic; communicative.

The development of the self-researcher-self-guinea pig-experimenter is guided by **principles**, methods, techniques and therapies, proposed by the *neoscience* or absorbed from other areas of knowledge, to be applied in self-research laboratories on conscientiological *campuses* and in everyday life. Here are 40 principles that exemplify the theory and practice of conscientiological self-research:

1. **Start.** Good self-research starts with a good *self-question*.

2. **Reach.** The conscientiologist always has a pen and paper at hand to make continuous notes.

3. **Registration.** If the experience draws your attention, but cannot be understood, it should be registered to be understood in the future.

4. **Detail.** "The smartest thing is to register everything in your research, even what currently seems insignificant or even silly"[1:401][Translation]. The overlooked detail will not be remembered to be understood.

5. **Confor** (*con*tent + *for*m). When recording on paper, prioritize the content and don't stick to the form. The first record is facilitated by acronyms, abbreviations, markings, and other personal resources to help shape the writing.

6. **Pen.** The best pen is the one that writes your records with minimal friction and effort, and even upside down, before getting

out of bed, avoiding the dispersion of subtle memories from extraphysical experiences. Felt tip pens or a rollerball with gel ink meet this requirement.

7. **Dictionary.** The expansion of the synonymic-antonymic-analogical-polyglottic brain dictionary facilitates the expression of ideas and experiences.

8. **Experience.** Self-research must be 1% theoretical and 99% practical, experiential[74:1099].

9. **Theorice** (*theory* + pract*ice*)**.** Theory allied to practice (self-experience) is the apex of self-knowledge. In theorical self-research, practice is superior to theory[1:470].

10. **Technique.** "The shortest path between theory (information) and practice (experience) is the technique"[121:41][Translation].

11. **Instrument.** The consciousness is the best research tool for the study of their own consciousness[1:660].

12. **Devices.** Holosomatic self-perception is superior to the measurements of laboratory research devices[1:409].

13. **Labcon** (*lab*oratory + *con*sciential)**.** The biggest self-research environment is the personal labcon.

14. **Compass.** Facts and parafacts guide the incessant self-research.

15. **Parapsychism.** Parapsychism allows for the concatenation of facts with parafacts. "The researcher-sensitive researches the integral consciousness"[168:1000][Translation].

16. **Signals.** The self-mastery of personal energetic and parapsychic signals qualifies self-research[201].

17. **Cosmovision.** The pluralization of research approaches develops the overall, generalist, multicultural, polyhedral and cosmovisiological view of the self-researcher.

18. **Participation.** Self-research, according to the consciential paradigm, is always participatory[168:935]. No consciousness acts alone in this or other dimensions.

19. **Priority.** Self-research is more of a priority than heteroresearch, or general research[202].

20. **Reverberation.** Strictly speaking, all research contains a percentage of self-research.

21. **Conscientiocentrism.** Every research topic is related to the consciousness. After all, there is no subject that is not related, from some perspective, to consciential manifestations.

22. **Interrelation.** The veteran self-researcher researches everything, all the time, relating the researched topics to the events surrounding them regarding the subtleties of everyday life[1:1248].

23. **Neoverpon.** The study of previously published findings, through a bibliographic review on the topic under investigation, prevents the researcher from *reinventing the wheel* and favors the emergence of neoverpons.

24. **Self-effort.** Research inspiration does not replace the perspiration of self-efforts during investigations[203]. "Genius is one percent inspiration and 99 percent perspiration" (Thomas Edison). "*The one who does not look, does not find*"[1:401][Translation].

25. **Autodidacticism.** The continuous practice of self-research improves the researcher. "*Nemo magister natus* (No one is born a master)"[1:402].

26. **Exemption.** Authentic self-research does not seek to please, impress, *make yourself look better than you are* or *improve your self-image.*

27. **Independence.** The independent self-researcher works without limiting their investigations to financial subsidies, academic titles, honors and decorations.

28. **Freedom.** The greater the relative freedom in investigations, the more authentic, reliable, and prolific the research will be.

29. **Cosmoethics.** Genuine self-research is cosmoethical in its motivation, in its *means* and in its *ends*.

30. **Purpose.** Self-research aims at self-evolution and the expansion of interassistantial maturity.

31. **Crisis.** Authentic self-research predisposes growth crises.

32. **Recin.** Intraconsciential recycling is the synthesis of self-research.

33. **Blind spot.** The consciousness always has some blind spot in which manifested traits escape their awareness.

34. **Intention.** Advanced self-research involves the assessment of self-intentionality.

35. **Thosenity.** The dissection of self-thosenity is inherent to the deepening of self-research.

36. **Exemplarism.** The continued self-effort to know themselves leads the self-researcher to being a *silent educator* of consciousnesses around them.

37. **Authorship.** The publication of verpons makes up the stages of productive self-research. "Any cosmoethical self-cognition is to be distributed for the benefit of humanity"[1:550][Translation].

38. **Completeness.** Strictly speaking, the self-research is only completed when the results are shared.

39. **Self-relay.** The publication of self-research findings favors a chain of assistantial actions by the lucid consciousness throughout their multiple human lives.

40. **Continuum.** After every horizon of research, there is always *a neo-horizon* to be explored. "*Doceri velle summa est eruditio*" (Wanting to learn is the supreme erudition)[1:547].

The **techniques**, methods and conscientiological therapies distributed throughout this book are just a small excerpt from the *pharmacopoeia*, or *valise of evolutionary tools*, proposed by the neoscience. The tools offered are intended to favor experimentation, but do not replace the researcher's own efforts to define their priorities, enable self-experience, develop neoverpons, mobilize recins and expand their free will and personal harmony, based on the *law of the greatest evolutionary effort*.

The *corpus* of Conscientiology is continuously expanding as a result of the investigations of self-research volunteers. Conscientiological neoconstructs stimulate the consciousness to explore other perspectives and reach **neoverpons** on the subjects studied.

Among the proposed research themes, we highlight the hypothesis of the existence of the **macrosoma,** an enhanced human body, that is *exceptional*, adapted and updated during the intermission, in order to favor the achievement of a specific existential program[204].

By deepening the understanding of their own health, the consciousness inevitably ends up studying **self-thosenity**. The thosene is the organizing principle of one's consciential manifestation, which regulates the homeostasis of the holosoma, from which health is structured. The anatomization of one's personal thosenity reveals the intimate reality of the consciousness, favors the liberation from self-imposed mental shackles and the expression of autonomy and free will.

Evolutionary effort expands the person's power over themselves, their **self-potentiality**, which begins to predominate in their personal manifestations in relation to the power exercised over others, characteristic of heteropotentiality. Self-potentiation means the relinquishing authority over other consciousnesses, while continuing to qualify the assistance provided to others[1:404].

Self-research accompanies the person who aspires to **neochallenges** along the ascending path of consciential evolution. The advances and metrics of the personal condition, from beginner to veteran, can be measured by the person themselves, using parameters and tools, such as the conscientiogram. The purpose is to broaden one's understanding of evolutionary responsibilities and motivate the person through the glimpse of new opportunities and realities.

Self-awareness and self-research are viewed as being the greatest challenge to qualifying self-care and developing self-sufficiency. In this way, science can come closer to the fundamental goal of improving the conditions of life and the world, based on the promotion of self-knowledge and self-awareness of each person. The **experienced** synergy of consciential self-research and recycling, collectively, is essential for the development of an increasingly fraternal and cosmoethical society.

Do you notice the *interactions* between your everyday ***self-care*** and your ***self-research***? Do you identify opportunities to *expand* your ***self-knowledge, self-awareness, and self-scientificity***? What benefits have you already achieved with your *self-research practices*?

References

1. Vieira, Waldo. *Dicionário de Argumentos da Conscienciologia*. Editares, 2014. 1572 p.
2. Arantes, Rosalba C et al. "Processo saúde-doença e promoção da saúde: aspectos históricos e conceituais". Revista de APS, v. 11, n. 2, 2008, pp. 189-198.
3. Sacconi, Luiz Antonio. *Grande Dicionário Sacconi: da língua portuguesa: comentado, crítico, enciclopédico*. São Paulo, 2010, p. 490.
4. Scliar, Moacyr. "História do conceito de saúde". Physis, v. 17, n. 1, 2007, pp. 29-41, https://www.scielo.br/j/physis/a/WNtwLvWQRFbscbz-CywV9wGq/abstract/?lang=en.
5. Collière, Marie-Françoise. *Promover a vida: da prática das mulheres de virtude aos cuidados de enfermagem*. Sindicato dos Enfermeiros Portugueses, 1989. 384 p.
6. Barros, Nelson Filice. *A Construção da Medicina Integrativa: um desafio para o campo da saúde*. Aderaldo & Rothschild, 2008. 311 p.
7. Queiroz, Marcus. S. O sentido do conceito de medicina alternativa e movimento vitalista: uma perspectiva teórica introdutória. In: Nascimento, Marilene Cabral (Org.). *As duas faces da montanha: estudos sobre medicina chinesa e acupuntura*. Hucitec, 2006.
8. Guedes, Carla Ribeiro et al. "A subjetividade como anomalia: contribuições epistemológicas para a crítica do modelo biomédico". Ciência e Saúde Coletiva, v. 11, n. 4, 2006, pp. 1093-1103. https://doi.org/10.1590/S1413-81232006000400030.
9. Luz, Madel Therezinha. "Cultura contemporânea e medicinas alternativas: novos paradigmas em saúde no fim do século XX". Physis, v. 7, n. 1, 1997, pp. 13-43. https://doi.org/10.1590/S0103-73311997000100002.
10. Zoboli, Elma Lourdes Campos Pavone. "Conferência Inicial: responsa-

bilidade para com a comunidade". Revista da Ordem dos Enfermeiros".
Revista Ordem dos Enfermeiros, n. 37, 2011, pp.7-17.

11. Mckenna Hugh. *Nursing theories and models*. Routlege, 2005. 256 p.

12. Meleis, Afaf Ibrahim. *Theoretical nursing: Development and progress*. 5th
ed. Lippincott Williams & Wilkins, 2011. 807 p.

13. Oliveira, Maria Amélia de Campos. "(Re)significando os projetos cui-
dativos da Enfermagem à luz das necessidades em saúde da população".
Revista Brasileira de Enfermagem, v. 65, n. 3, 2012, pp. 401-405, 2012.
http://dx.doi.org/10.1590/S0034-71672012000300002.

14. Souza, Luis Eugênio Portela Fernandes. Saúde Pública ou Saúde Coletiva? Espaço para Saúde, v. 15, n. 4, 2014, pp. 7-21. http://dx.doi.or-
g/10.22421/15177130-2014v15n4p7.

15. Nunes, Everardo Duarte. "Saúde Coletiva: Revisitando a sua História e
os Cursos de Pós-Graduação". Ciência e Saúde Coletiva, v. 1, n. 1, 1996,
pp. 55-69. https://doi.org/10.1590/1413-812319961101392014.

16. Mello, Guilherme A. "Quando os paradigmas mudam na saúde pública: o que muda na história?" História, Ciências, Saúde – Manguinhos,
2017, v. 24, n. 2, 2017, pp. 499-517. https://www.redalyc.org/articulo.
oa?id=386151662013.

17. World Health Organization. *Constitution of the World Health Organization*. WHO, 1946. https://apps.who.int/gb/bd/PDF/bd47/EN/consti-
tution-en.pdf?ua=1.

18. World Health Organization. *Ottawa Charter for Heath Promotion, 1986*.
https://www.euro.who.int/__data/assets/pdf_file/0004/129532/Ot-
tawa_Charter.pdf

19. Chiesa, Anna Maria et al. "A formação de profissionais da saúde: apren-
dizagem significativa à luz da promoção da saúde". Cogitare Enfermagem,
v. 12, n. 2, pp. 236-240, 2007. http://dx.doi.org/10.5380/ce.v12i2.9829.

20. Haeser, Laura de Macedo et al. "Considerações sobre a autonomia e a
promoção da saúde". Physis, v. 22, n. 2, pp. 605-620, 2012. https://doi.
org/10.1590/S0103-73312012000200011.

21. Puttini, Rodolfo Franco et al. "Modelos explicativos em saúde coletiva:
abordagem biopsicossocial e auto-organização". Physis, v. 20, n. 3, pp.
753-767, 2010. https://doi.org/10.1590/S0103-73312010000300004.

22. Campos, Gastão Wagner de Souza. Subjetividade e Administração de
Pessoal: considerações sobre modos de gerenciar o trabalho em equipes
de saúde. In: Merhy, E. E.; Onocko R. (Orgs.). *Agir em saúde: um desafio
para o público*. Hucitec, 2006, pp. 229-266.

23. Zoboli, Elma Lourdes Campos Pavone et al. O cuidado de enfermagem
em saúde coletiva. In: Soares, Cassia Baldini; Campos, Célia Maria Sival-

li. (Orgs.). *Fundamentos de Saúde Coletiva e o Cuidado de Enfermagem.* Manole 2013, v. 1, p. 244-264.

24. Schveitzer, Mariana Cabral. *Concepções de saúde e cuidado de práticas integrativas/complementares e humanizadoras na Atenção Básica: uma revisão sistemática.* [Tese]. Escola de Enfermagem da Universidade de São Paulo - EEUSP, 2015. 267 p. https://www.teses.usp.br/teses/disponiveis/7/7141/tde-13052015-103633/pt-br.php.

25. Brasil. Ministério da Saúde. Secretaria de Atenção à Saúde. Departamento de Atenção Básica. *PNPIC Política nacional de práticas integrativas e complementares no SUS: atitude de ampliação de acesso.* 2nd ed. Ministério da Saúde, 96 p, 2015. http://bvsms.saude.gov.br/bvs/publicacoes/politica_nacional_praticas_integrativas_complementares_2ed.pdf.

26. Brasil. Ministério da Saúde. Secretaria de Atenção à Saúde. Núcleo Técnico da Política Nacional de Humanização. *HumanizaSUS: documento base para gestores e trabalhadores do SUS.* Ministério da Saúde, 74 p, 2006. https://bvsms.saude.gov.br/bvs/publicacoes/humanizasus_documento_gestores_trabalhadores_sus.pdf.

27. Zoboli, Elma Lourdes Campos Pavone. "Bioética e atenção básica: para uma clínica ampliada, uma bioética amplificada". O Mundo da Saúde, v. 33, n. 2, 2009, pp. 195-204.

28. Scholze, Alessandro da Silva et al. Trabalho em saúde e a implantação do acolhimento na atenção primária à saúde: afeto, empatia ou alteridade? Interface (Botucatu), v. 13, n. 31, 2009, pp. 303-314. https://doi.org/10.1590/S1414-32832009000400006.

29. Larson, James S. "The conceptualization of health". Medical care research and review: MCRR, v. 56, n. 2, 1990, pp. 123-36. https://doi.org/10.1177/107755879905600201.

30. Tarride, Mario Ivan. *Saúde Pública: uma complexidade anunciada.* FIOCRUZ, 1998. 112 p.

31. Pinheiro, Roseni; Luz, Madel Therezinha. *Modelos ideais x práticas eficazes: um desencontro entre gestores e clientela nos serviços de saúde.* UERJ/IMS, 1999. 23 p. (Studies in Collective Health, 191).

32. Luz, Madel Therezinha. Prefácio. In: Nascimento M C. (Org.). *As duas faces da montanha: estudos sobre medicina chinesa e acupuntura.* Hucitec, 2006.

33. Luz, Madel Terezinha; Barros, Nelson Filice. (Orgs.) *Racionalidades Médicas e Práticas Integrativas em Saúde: estudos teóricos e empíricos.* CEPESC-IMS-UERJ, Abrasco, 2012.

34. World Health Organization. *Primary health care: report of the International Conference on Primary Health Care, Alma-Ata, USSR, 6-12 September 1978.* WHO, 1978. https://apps.who.int/iris/handle/10665/39228.

35. World Health Organization. *Traditional Medicine Strategy: 2014-2023*. WHO, 2013. https://apps.who.int/iris/bitstream/handle/10665/92455/9789241506090_eng.pdf?sequence=1.

36. World Health Organization. *WHO Global Atlas of Traditional, Complementary and Alternative medicine*. WHO, 2019. https://apps.who.int/iris/handle/10665/43108.

37. World Health Organization. *General Guidelines for Methodologies on Research and Evaluation of Traditional Medicine*. WHO, 2000. 80 p. https://apps.who.int/iris/bitstream/handle/10665/66783/WHO_EDM_TRM_2000.1.pdf?sequence=1/.

38. World Health Organization. *WHO Global Report on traditional and complementary medicine 2019*. WHO, 2019. 228 p. https://www.who.int/traditional-complementary-integrative-medicine/WhoGlobalReportOnTraditionalAndComplementaryMedicine2019.pdf?ua=1.

39. Frass, Michael et al. "Use and acceptance of complementary and alternative medicine among the general population and medical personnel: a systematic review". Ochsner Journal, v.12, n. 1, 2012, pp. 45-56. https://pubmed.ncbi.nlm.nih.gov/22438782/.

40. Cunha, Gustavo Tenório. *A construção da clínica ampliada na atenção básica*. Hucitec, 2005.

41. Almeida, Verônica. *Oferta de PICS cresce na atenção primária e especializada*. ObservaPICS; c2019. http://observapics.fiocruz.br/oferta-de-pics-cresce-na-atencao-primaria-e-especializada/.

42. Brasil. Ministério da Saúde. Portaria n. 849, de 21 de março de 2017. *Inclui a Arteterapia, Ayurveda, Biodança, Dança Circular, Meditação, Musicoterapia, Naturopatia, Osteopatia, Quiropraxia, Reflexoterapia, Reiki, Shantala, Terapia Comunitária Integrativa e Yoga à Política Nacional de Práticas Integrativas e Complementares*. Diário Oficial da União, 27 mar. 2017. sec. 1, p. 68. http://bit.ly/2OgDsbY.

43. *I Congresso Internacional de Práticas Integrativas e Complementares e Saúde Pública*. Rio de Janeiro, 12 to 15 March, 2018. http://aps.saude.gov.br/congrepics/#!/.

44. Brasil. Ministério da Saúde. *Glossário Temático de Práticas Integrativas e Complementares*. Ministério da Saúde, 2018. 181p. https://portalarquivos2.saude.gov.br/images/pdf/2018/marco/12/glossario-tematico.pdf.

45. Brieghel-Muller Gunna. *Eutonia e Relaxamento*. Summus, 1998. 107p.

46. Kabat-Zinn, Jon. *Wherever you go, there you are: mindfulness meditation*. 1st ed. Hyperion. 1994. 277p.

47. Fredrickson, Barbara. *Positividade: Descubra a força das emoções positivas, supere a negatividade e viva plenamente*. 1st ed. Roxo. 2009. 272p.

48. Seligman, Martin E. P. *Flourish: A New Understanding of Happiness and Wellbeing: The practical guide to using positive psychology to make you happier and healthier*. Nicholas Brealey Publishing, 2011. 370 p.

49. Achor, Shawn. *The Happiness Advantage: The Seven Principles of Positive Psychology That Fuel Success and Performance at Work*. Crown Business, 2012. 256 p.

50. Chamine, Shirzad. *Inteligência positiva: por que só 20% das equipes e dos indivíduos alcançam seu verdadeiro potencial e como você pode alcançar o seu*. Fontanar, 2013. 228 p.

51. Tanaka, Nobutaka. O que é spiral taping. 4th ed. Spiral Taping do Brasil, 2003.

52. Dias, Álvaro Machado. "Tendências do neurofeedback em psicologia: revisão sistemática". Psicologia em estudo. v. 15, n. 4, pp. 811-820. https://doi.org/10.1590/S1413-73722010000400017.

53. Servan-Schreiber, David. *The Instinct to Heal: Curing Depression, Anxiety and Stress Without Drugs and Without Talk Therapy*. Rodale Press, 2005. 288 p.

54. Otani, Márcia Aparecida Padovan; Barros, Nelson Filice de. "A Medicina Integrativa e a construção de um novo modelo na saúde". Ciência saúde coletiva, v. 16, n. 3, 2011, pp. 1801-1811. https://doi.org/10.1590/S1413-81232011000300016.

55. Teixeira, Marcus Zulian. "Bases psiconeurofisiológicas do fenômeno placebo-nocebo: evidências científicas que valorizam a humanização da relação médico-paciente". Revista da Associação Medica Brasileira, v. 55, n. 1, 2009, pp. 13-18.

56. Chao, Maria T et al. "Disclosure of complementary and alternative medicine to conventional medical providers: variation by race/ethnicity and type of CAM". Journal of the National Medical Association, v. 100, n. 11, 2008, pp. 1341, https://doi.org/10.1016/s0027-9684(15)31514-5.

57. Singer, Charles and Underwood, E. Ashworth. *Short History of Medicine*. 2nd ed. Oxford University Press, 1962. 854 p.

58. Chiesa, Gustavo Ruiz. *Além do que se vê: magnetismos, ectoplasmas e paracirurgias*. Multifoco, 2016.

59. Hippocrates. On the Sacred Disease. In: *Works by Hippocrates*. Translated by Francis Adams. http://classics.mit.edu/Hippocrates/sacred.html.

60. Rezende, Joffre Marcondes. À sombra do plátano: crônicas de história da medicina.: Editora Unifesp, 2009. Capítulo: dos quatro humores às quatro bases. pp. 49-53, http://books.scielo.org/id/8kf92/pdf/rezende-9788561673635-05.pdf.

61. Martins, Roberto de Andrade et al. *Contágio: história da prevenção das doenças transmissíveis*. Moderna, 1997, http://webcache.googleusercontent.com/search?q=cache:http://www.ghtc.usp.br/Contagio/intro.html&gws_rd=cr&dcr=0&ei=Z8D9WeGfPMmtwATu1IuIBw.

62. Donatelli, Marisa Carneiro de Oliveira Franco. "Descartes e os médicos". Scientiæ studia, v. 1, n. 3, 2003, pp. 323-36.

63. Teixeira, Marcus Zulian. "Antropologia Médica Vitalista: uma ampliação ao entendimento do processo de adoecimento humano". Revista Médica (São Paulo), v. 96, n. 3, 2017, pp. 145-58.

64. Schneider, João Ricardo. *História do Parapsiquismo*. Editares, 2018, pp. 420- 421.

65. Vieira, Waldo. Conscienciologia [verbete]. In: Vieira, Waldo (Org.). *Enciclopédia da Conscienciologia*. 9th ed. Digital. Version 9. Editares, 2018, https://editares.org.br/livro/enciclopedia-da-conscienciologia-9a-edicao/.

66. Vieira, Waldo. Cronologia da Projeciologia [verbete]. In: Vieira, Waldo (Org.). *Enciclopédia da Conscienciologia*. 9th ed. Digital. Version 9. Editares, 2018. https://editares.org.br/livro/enciclopedia-da-conscienciologia-9a-edicao/

67. Vieira, Waldo. *Projectiology: a panorama of experiences of the consciousness outside the human body*. Editares, 2016. 1210 p.

68. Cordioli, Cesar. *Conscienciologia: Breve Introdução à Ciência da Consciência*. Foz do Iguaçu: Editares, 2019.

69. Schveitzer, Fernanda Cabral. Saúde Consciencial [verbete]. In: Vieira, Waldo (Org.). *Enciclopédia da Conscienciologia*. 9th ed. Digital. Version 9. Editares, 2018. https://editares.org.br/livro/enciclopedia-da-conscienciologia-9a-edicao/.

70. Vieira, Waldo. Anticura [verbete]. In: Vieira, Waldo (Org.). *Enciclopédia da Conscienciologia*. 9th ed. Digital. Version 9. Editares, 2018. https://editares.org.br/livro/enciclopedia-da-conscienciologia-9a-edicao/.

71. Vieira, Waldo. *Léxico de Ortopensatas*. Editares, 2014. 1507 p.

72. Machado, Cesar. *Proatividade Evolutiva*. Editares, 2013. 440 p.

73. Duncan, Bruce B et al. *Medicina ambulatorial: condutas de atenção primária baseadas em evidências*. 3rd ed. Artmed, 2006. 116 p.

74. Vieira, Waldo. *Homo sapiens reurbanisatus*. 3rd ed. Associação Internacional do Centro de Altos Estudos da Conscienciologia – CEAEC, 2005. 1584 p.

75. Vieira, Waldo. *700 Conscientiology Experiments*. Editares, 2016. 1056 p.

76. Rosenfield, Denis Lerrer. Vida e Obra. In: Descartes R. *Discurso do Método*. L&PM, 2005.

77. Japiassú, Hilton; Marcondes, Danilo. *Dicionário Básico de Filosofia*. 3rd ed. Jorge Zahar, 1996.

78. Kuhn, Thomas S. *The Structure of Scientific Revolutions*. 2nd ed. University of Chicago Press, 1970.

79. Silveira, Rosemari Monteiro Castilho Foggiatto; Bazzo, Walter. "Ciência, tecnologia e suas relações sociais: a percepção de geradores de tecnologia e suas implicações na educação tecnológica". Ciência & Educação (Bauru), v. 15, n. 3, 2009, pp. 681-694. https://doi.org/10.1590/S1516-73132009000300014.

80. Minayo, Maria Cecília de S; Sanchez, Odécio. "Quantitativo-Qualitativo: oposição ou complementaridade"? Caderno de Saúde Pública, v. 9, n, 3, 1993, pp. 239-262. https://www.scielo.br/pdf/csp/v9n3/02.pdf.

81. Barreto, Maurício L. "O conhecimento científico e tecnológico como evidência para políticas e atividades regulatórias em saúde". Ciência saúde coletiva, v. 9, n. 2, 2004, pp. 329-338. https://doi.org/10.1590/S1413-81232004000200010

82. Lawn, Chris. *Compreender Gadamer*. Vozes, 2007. 208 p.

83. Pinzani, Alessandro. *Habermas: Introdução*. Artmed, 2009. 160 p.

84. Ayres, José Ricardo de Carvalho Mesquita. "Sujeito, intersubjetividade e práticas de saúde". Ciência saúde coletiva, v. 6, n. 1, 2001, pp. 63-72. http://dx.doi.org/10.1590/S1413-81232001000100005.

85. Habermas, Jürgen. *Teoría de la acción comunicativa*. Taurus, 1987. 516 p.

86. Bettine, Marco. A *Teoria do Agir Comunicativo de Jürgen Habermas: bases conceituais*. Edições EACH, 2021. http://www.livrosabertos.sibi.usp.br/portaldelivrosUSP/catalog/book/587.

87. Minayo, Maria Ceília de S. *O Desafio do Conhecimento: pesquisa qualitativa em saúde*. 8th ed. Hucitec, 2004. 416 p.

88. Prado, Marta Lenise; Souza, Maria Lourdes; Carraro, Thelma Elisa. *Investigación cualitativa en enfermería: contexto y bases conceptuales*. OPAS, 2008. (Serie PALTEX Salud y Sociedad, 2000; 9). https://iris.paho.org/handle/10665.2/51581.

89. Turato, Egberto Ribeiro. "Métodos qualitativos e quantitativos na área da saúde: definições, diferenças e seus objetos de pesquisa." Revista de Saúde Pública, v. 39, n. 3, 2005, pp. 507-514. https://doi.org/10.1590/S0034-89102005000300025.

90. Rolfe, Gary. "Validity, trustworthiness and rigor: quality and the idea of qualitative research". Journal of Advanced Nursing, v. 53, n. 3, 2006, pp. 304-310.

91. Reeves, Scott et al. *Why use theories in qualitative research?* BMJ, v. 337, 2008, pp. 631-634.

92. Creswell, John W. A *Concise Introduction to Mixed Methods Research*. Thousand Oaks, 2015.

93. Rogers, Everett M. *Diffusion of Innovations*. 5th ed. Free Press, 2004. 574 p.

94. Chamberlain, Paul. "Knowledge is not everything." Design for Health, v. 4, n. 1, 2020, pp. 1-3. https://doi.org/10.1080/24735132.2020.1731203.

95. Egger, Matthias et al. (Orgs.). *Systematic Reviews in Health Care: Meta-analysis in context*. BMJ books, 2001.

96. Grant, Maria J; Booth, Andrew. "A typology of reviews: an analysis of 14 review types and associated methodologies". Health Information & Libraries Journal, v. 26, n. 2, 2009, pp. 91-108. https://doi.org/10.1111/j.1471-1842.2009.00848.x.

97. O'Leary, Bethan C et al. "Evidence maps and evidence gaps: evidence review mapping as a method for collating and appraising evidence reviews to inform research and policy". Environmental Evidence, v. 6, n. 19, 2017, pp. 19. https://doi.org/10.1186/s13750-017-0096-9.

98. Morris, Zoe. S; Wooding, Steven; Grant, Jonathan. "The answer is 17 years, what is the question: understanding time lags in translational research". Journal of the Royal Society of Medicine, v. 104, n. 12, 2011, pp. 510-520. https://doi.org/10.1258/jrsm.2011.110180.

99. Gnatta, Juliana Rizzo et al. "Aromatherapy and nursing: historical and theoretical Conception". Revista da Escola de Enfermagem USP, v. 50, n. 1, 2016, pp. 127-133, 2016. http://dx.doi.org/10.1590/S0080-623420160000100017.

100. Svenaus, Fredrik. "Hermeneutics of medicine in the wake of Gadamer: the issue of phronesis". Theoretical Medicine and Bioethics, v. 24, n. 5, 2003, pp. 407-431. https://doi.org/10.1023/b:meta.0000006935.10835.b2.

101. Salles, Léia Fortes; Kurebayashi, Leonice Fumiko Sato; Silva, Maria Julia Paes. As práticas complementares e a Enfermagem. In: Salles, L F; Silva, M J P. (Orgs.). *Enfermagem e as práticas complementares em saúde*. Yendis, 2011, pp. 1-18.

102. Tesser, Charles Dalcanale; Sousa, Islândia Maria Carvalho de. "Atenção primária, atenção psicossocial, práticas integrativas e complementares e suas afinidades eletivas". Saude e sociedade, v. 21, n. 2, 2012, pp. 336-350. http://dx.doi.org/10.1590/S0104-12902012000200008.

103. Pierce Beverly A et al. "Physician Perspectives on Comparative Effectiveness Research: Implications for Practice-based Evidence". Global Advances in Health and Medicine, v. 1, n. 4, 2012, pp. 32-6, https://doi.org/10.7453/gahmj.2012.1.4.004.

104. Dossett, Michelle L; Fricchione, Gregory, L; Benson, Herbert B. "A New Era for Mind-Body Medicine". New England Journal of Medicine, v. 382, n. 15, 2020, pp. 1390–1391. https://doi.org/10.1056/NEJMp1917461.

105. Curi, Luciano Marcos; Santos, Roberto Carlos dos. "Ludwik Fleck e a análise sociocultural da(s) ciência(s)". História ciências saúde-Mangui-

nhos, v. 18, n. 4, 2011, pp. 1169-1173, 2011. https://doi.org/10.1590/S0104-59702011000400013.

106. Schveitzer, Mariana Cabral. *Estilos de Pensamento em Educação em Enfermagem: uma análise da produção científica das regiões Norte, Nordeste e Centro-oeste do Brasil.* Dissertação (Mestrado em Enfermagem). Centro de Ciencias da Saúde da Universidade Federal de Santa Catarina - UFSC, 2010, 123 p. https://repositorio.ufsc.br/xmlui/handle/123456789/94648.

107. Cutolo, Luiz Roberto Agea. *Estilo de pensamento em educação médica: um estudo do currículo do curso de graduação em medicina da UFSC.* Tese (Doutorado em Educação) - Centro de Ciências da Educação, Universidade Federal de Santa Catarina, 2001.

108. Fleck, Ludwik. *Genesis and Development of a Scientific Fact.* University of Chicago Press, 1992. 203 p.

109. Löwy, Ilana. "Introduction: Ludwick Fleck's epistemology of medicine and biomedical sciences". Studies in History and Philosophy of Science Part C: Studies in History and Biological and Biomedical Science, v. 35, n. 3, 2004, pp. 437-445.

110. Pereira, Isabel Brasil. *Interdisciplinaridade.* Dicionário da Educação Profissional em Saúde (on-line). Escola Politécnica de Saúde Joaquim Venâncio. 2009. http://www.sites.epsjv.fiocruz.br/dicionario/verbetes/int.html.

111. Peduzzi, Marina. *Trabalho em Equipe.* Dicionário da Educação Profissional em Saúde (on-line). Escola Politécnica de Saúde Joaquim Venâncio. 2009.

112. Leite, Hernande. "Metodologia de Autopesquisa". Conscientia, v. 17, n. 2, 2013, pp. 163-170, 2013.

113. Schveitzer, Mariana Cabral. "Consciousness Research and psychic phenomena. Interview with Dean Radin (IONS)". Interparadigmas, ano 5, n. 5, 2017, pp. 329-332. https://www.interparadigmas.org.br/?page_id=350.

114. Queiroz, Maria Isaura Pereira. "Relatos orais: do "indizível" ao "dizível". Ciência e Cultura, v. 39, n. 3, 1987, pp. 272- 286.

115. Hoga, Luiza Akiko Komura; Pereira, Priscila Faria. Paradigmas de pesquisa. In: Hoga, Luiza Akiko Komura; Borges, Ana Luiza Vilela. (Orgs.). *Pesquisa empírica em saúde: guia prático para iniciantes.* EEUSP, 2016, p. 13-21.

116. De Castro, Thiago Gomes; Gomes, William Barbosa. "Aplicações do método fenomenológico à pesquisa em psicologia: tradições e tendências". Estudos de Psicologia, v. 28, n. 2, 2011, pp. 153-171.

117. Ayres, José Ricardo de Carvalho Mesquita. "Para comprender el sentido prático de las acciones de salud: contribuciones da la hermenéutica filosófica". Salud Colectiva, v. 4, n. 2, 2008, pp. 159-172.

118. Mota, Tathiana. *Intermissive Course: Have you prepared yourself for the challenges of human life?* Editares, 2019. 212 p.

119. Vieira, Waldo. Antepassado de si mesmo [verbete]. In: Vieira, Waldo (Org.). *Enciclopédia da Conscienciologia*. 9th ed. Digital. Version 9. Editares, 2018. https://editares.org.br/livro/enciclopedia-da-conscienciologia-9a-edicao/.

120. Luz, Marcelo da. *Where does religion end?* Editares, 2017. 485 p.

121. Balona, Malú. *Autocura através da reconciliação: estudo prático sobre afetividade*. Editares, 2015. 369 p.

122. Louzada, Rita de Cássia Ramos; Silva Filho, João Ferreira da. "Tornar-se pesquisador: a escolha profissional como um processo". Psicologia em Estudo, v. 13, n. 4, 2008, pp. 753-760. https://dx.doi.org/10.1590/S1413-73722008000400013.

123. Zaslavski, Alexandre. "Autoexperimentação Consciencial: O Método Científico Conscienciológico". Conscientia, v. 23, n. 3, 2019, pp. 147-158.

124. Fertonani, Hosanna Pattrig et al. "Modelo assistencial em saúde: conceitos e desafios para a atenção básica brasileira". Ciência saúde coletiva, v. 20, n. 6, 2015, pp. 1869-1878. https://doi.org/10.1590/1413-81232015206.13272014.

125. Almeida, Maria Cecília Puntel; Rocha, Juan Stuardo Yazlle. *O saber de enfermagem e sua dimensão prática*. Cortez, 1986.

126. Ayres, José Ricardo C. M. *Cuidado: trabalho e interação nas práticas de saúde*. ABRASCO, 2009. (Coleção Clássicos para Integralidade em Saúde). 143 p. https://www.cepesc.org.br/wp-content/uploads/2013/08/miolo-livro-ricardo.pdf.

127. Malta, Deborah Carvalho; Merhy, Emerson Elias. "A micropolítica do processo de trabalho em saúde: revendo alguns conceitos". Reme: Revista Mineira de Enfermagem, v. 7, n. 1, 2003, pp. 61-66. https://www.reme.org.br/artigo/detalhes/786.

128. Meier, Marineli Joaguim.; Cianciarullo, Tamara Iwanow. "Tecnologia: um conceito em construção para o trabalhador em saúde". Texto & Contexto Enfermagem, v. 11, n. 1, 2002, pp. 31-49, 2002.

129. Gonçalves, Ricardo Bruno Mendes. *Tecnologia e organização social das práticas de saúde: características tecnológicas de processo de trabalho na Rede Estadual de Centros de Saúde de São Paulo*. Hucitec, 1994. 278 p. (Saúde em Debate, 76).

130. Merhy, Emerson Elias; Onocko, Rosana. *Agir em saúde: um desafio para o público*. Hucitec, 1997.

131. Merhy, Emerson Elias. Saúde: a cartográfica do trabalho vivo em ato. Hucitec, 2007.

132. Garbois, Júlia Arêas; Sodré, Francis; Dalbello-Araujo, Maristela. "Da noção de determinação social à de determinantes sociais da saúde". Saúde debate, v. 41, n. 112, 2017, pp. 63-76. https://doi.org/10.1590/0103-1104201711206.

133. Ogata, Márcia Niituma. *Concepções de saúde e doença: estudo das representações sociais de profissionais da saúde*. 2000. Tese (Doutorado em Enfermagem) - Escola de Enfermagem de Ribeirão Preto da Universidade de São Paulo, 2000.

134. Ospina, Naykky Singh et al. "Eliciting the Patient's Agenda- Secondary Analysis of Recorded Clinical Encounters". Journal of General Internal Medicine, v. 34, n. 1, 2019, pp. 36-40. https://doi.org/10.1007/s11606-018-4540-5.

135. Mitchell, Rebecca et al. Review: "Toward Realizing the Potential of Diversity in Composition of Psychosocial Dynamics of Interprofessional Collaboration Interprofessional Health Care Teams: An Examination of the Cognitive and Psychosocial Dynamics of Interprofessional Collaboration". Medical Care Research and Review: MCRR, v. 67, n. 1, 2010, pp. 3–26, 2010. https://pubmed.ncbi.nlm.nih.gov/19605620/.

136. Recthin, Sheldon M. "A conceptual framework for interprofessional and co-managed care". Academic medicine: journal of the Association of American Medical College, v. 83, n. 10, 2008, pp. 929–33, 2008. https://doi.org/10.1097/ACM.0b013e3181850b4b.

137. Sangaleti, Carine et al. "Experiences and shared meaning of teamwork and interprofessional collaboration among health care professionals in primary health care settings: a systematic review". JBI database of systematic reviews and implementation reports, v. 15, n. 11, 2017, pp. 2723-2788. https://doi.org/10.11124/JBISRIR-2016-003016.

138. Mccallin, Antoinette M. "Interdisciplinary researching: exploring the opportunities and risks of working together". Nursing & Health Sciences, v. 8, n. 2, 2006, pp. 88-94. https://doi.org/10.1111/j.1442-2018.2006.00257.x.

139. Hsiao, Jony; Schveitzer, Mariana Cabral; Germani, Ana Claudia. Colaboração Interprofissional para oferta de Práticas Integrativas na Atenção Primária à Saúde. In: Gouveia, Gisele Damian Antonio (Org.). *Práticas Integrativas em Saúde: aprendizado em serviço*. Paco Editorial, 2019, p. 67-81.

140. Word Health Organization. *Framework for Action on Interprofessional Education & Collaborative Practice*. WHO, 2010. 64 p. https://apps.who.int/iris/bitstream/handle/10665/70185/WHO_HRH_HPN_10.3_eng.pdf?sequence=1.

141. Agreli, Heloise Fernandes; Peduzzi, Marina; Silva, Mariana Charantola. "Atenção centrada no paciente na prática interprofissional colaborativa". Interface (Botucatu), v. 20, n. 59, 2016, pp. 905-916. https://doi.org/10.1590/1807-57622015.0511.

142. Schveitzer, Mariana Cabral. Acolhimento Universal [verbete]. In: Vieira, Waldo (Org.). *Enciclopédia da Conscienciologia*. 9th ed. Digital. Version 9. Editares, 2018. https://editares.org.br/livro/enciclopedia-da-conscienciologia-9a-edicao/.

143. Tesser, Charles Dalcanale; Luz, Madel Therezinha. Racionalidades médicas e integralidade. Ciência saúde coletiva, v. 13, n. 1, 2008, pp. 195-206, 2008. http://dx.doi.org/10.1590/S1413-81232008000100024.

144. Foucault, Michel. *Vigiar e punir: nascimento da prisão*. 29th ed. Translation by de Raquel Ramalhete. Vozes, 2004, p. 125-52.

145. Brasil. Ministério da Saúde. Secretaria de Atenção à Saúde. *Núcleo Técnico da Política Nacional de Humanização. Clínica ampliada, equipe de referência projeto terapêutico singular*. 2nd ed. Ministério da Saúde, 2008. 60 p. http://bvsms.saude.gov.br/bvs/publicacoes/clinica_ampliada_equipe_projeto_2ed.pdf.

146. Rogers, Carl. R. *On Becoming a Person: A Therapist's View of Psychotherapy*. 6th ed. Houghton Mifflin, 1995. 420 p.

147. Safder, Taimur. "The Name of the Dog". The New England journal of medicine, v. 379, n. 14, 2018, pp. 1299-1301. https://dx.doi.org/10.1056/NEJMp1806388.

148. Ayres, José Ricardo de Carvalho Mesquita. "O cuidado, os modos de ser (do) humano e as práticas de saúde". Saúde Sociedade, v. 13, n. 3, 2004, pp. 16-29. http://dx.doi.org/10.1590/S0104-12902004000300003.

149. Brasil. Ministério da Saúde. Secretaria de Atenção à Saúde. Portaria n.1083, de 2 de outubro de 2012. *Aprova o protocolo clínico e diretrizes terapêuticas da dor crônica*. Diário Oficial da União, n. 214, de 05 de nov. 2002, sec, 1 p. 82. http://bvsms.saude.gov.br/bvs/saudelegis/sas/2012/prt1083_02_10_2012.html.

150. De Souza, Juliana Barcellos et al. "Prevalence of Chronic Pain, Treatments, Perception, and Interference on Life Activities: Brazilian Population-Based Survey". Pain research & management, 2017, pp. 4643830. https://dx.doi.org/10.1155/2017/4643830.

151. World Health Organization. *Acupuncture: review and analysis of reports on controlled clinical trials*. WHO, 2002. 81 p. http://digicollection.org/hss/en/d/Js4926e/.

152. Mambretti Giorgio; Séraphin Jean. *La medicina patas arriba ¿Y si Hamer tuviera razón?* Obelisco, 2002. 160 p.

153. Cardoso, Hugo Ferrari et al. "Síndrome de burnout: análise da literatura nacional entre 2006 e 2015". Revista Psicologia Organizações e Trabalho, v. 17, n. 2, 2017, pp. 121-128, 2017. https://dx.doi.org/10.17652/rpot/2017.2.12796.

154. Takimoto, Nário; Almeida, Roberto. "Conscienciotherapy: A Clinical Experience of the Nucleus of Integral Assistance for the Consciousness". Journal of Conscientiology, v. 4, n. 15S, 2002, pp. 21-41.

155. Takimoto, Nário. "Principios Teáticos da Consciencioterapia". Journal of Conscientiology, v. 9, n, 33S, 2006, pp. 11-28.

156. Estermann, Regina. Ciclo autoconsciencioterápico [verbete]. In: Vieira, Waldo (Org.). *Enciclopédia da Conscienciologia*. 9th ed. Digital. Version 9. Editares, 2018. https://editares.org.br/livro/enciclopedia-da-conscienciologia-9a-edicao/.

157. Gesing, Alzira. "Autopesquisa Conscienciométrica aplicada à interassistencialidade Parapedagógica". Revista de Parapedagogia, 2012, pp. 69-80.

158. Guimarães, Tânia. "Consciential evolutionary dynamics". Interparadigmas, v. 1, n.1, 2013, pp. 89-101. https://www.interparadigmas.org.br/?page_id=7.

159. Burkhard, Gudrun. *Tomar a vida nas próprias mãos: como trabalhar na própria biografia o conhecimento das leis gerais do desenvolvimento humano*. 4th ed. Antroposófica, 2010.

160. Antunes, Luiz Fernando. Antiadicção [verbete]. In: Vieira, Waldo (Org.). *Enciclopédia da Conscienciologia*. 9th ed. Digital. Version 9. Editares, 2018. https://editares.org.br/livro/enciclopedia-da-conscienciologia-9a--edicao/.

161. Arakaki, Kátia. *Antibagulhismo energético*. Editares, 2015. 190 p.

162. Arakaki, Kátia. Antibagulhismo Energético [verbete]. In: Vieira, Waldo (Org.). *Enciclopédia da Conscienciologia*. 9th ed. Digital. Version 9. Editares, 2018. https://editares.org.br/livro/enciclopedia-da-conscienciologia--9a-edicao/.

163. Vieira, Waldo. Autocura [verbete]. In: Vieira, Waldo (Org.). *Enciclopédia da Conscienciologia*. 9th ed. Digital. Version 9. Editares, 2018. https://editares.org.br/livro/enciclopedia-da-conscienciologia-9a-edicao/.

164. Musskopf, Tony. Autenticidade Consciencial [verbete] In: Vieira, Waldo (Org.). *Enciclopédia da Conscienciologia*. 9th ed. Digital. Version 9. Edita-

res, 2018. https://editares.org.br/livro/enciclopedia-da-conscienciologia-
-9a-edicao/.

165. Vieira, Waldo. Rotina Útil [verbete]. In: Vieira, Waldo (Org.). *Enciclopédia da Conscienciologia*. 9th ed. Digital. Version 9. Editares, 2018. https://editares.org.br/livro/enciclopedia-da-conscienciologia-9a-edicao/.

166. Vieira, Waldo. *100 testes da conscienciometria*. Instituto Internacional de Projeciologia e Conscienciologia, 1997. 232 p.

167. Couto, Cirleine. *Contrapontos do Parapsiquismo: Superação do Assédio Interconsciencial Rumo à Desassedialidade Permanente Total*. Editares, 2010. 212 p.

168. Vieira, Waldo. *Homo sapiens pacificus*. 3rd ed. Associação Internacional do Centro de Altos Estudos da Conscienciologia – CEAEC; Editares, 2007. 1584 p.

169. Martins, Eduardo. Padrão Homeostático de Referência [verbete]. In: Vieira, Waldo (Org.). *Enciclopédia da Conscienciologia*. 9th ed. Digital. Version 9. Editares, 2018. https://editares.org.br/livro/enciclopedia-da-conscienciologia-9a-edicao/.

170. Silva, Irene de Jesus et al. "Cuidado, autocuidado e cuidado de si: uma compreensão paradigmática para o cuidado de enfermagem". Revista da Escola de Enfermagem da USP, v. 43, n. 3, 2009, pp. 697-703. https://doi.org/10.1590/S0080-62342009000300028.

171. Vieira, Waldo. *Penta Manual: personal energetic task*. 3rd ed. Editares, 2016. 141 p.

172. Kauati, Adriana. Síndrome do Impostor [verbete]. In: Vieira, Waldo (Org.). *Enciclopédia da Conscienciologia*. 9th ed. Digital. Version 9. Editares, 2018. https://editares.org.br/livro/enciclopedia-da-conscienciologia-9a-edicao/.

173. Dahlke, Rüdiger; Dethlefsen, T. *The Healing Power of Illness: understanding what your symptoms are telling you*. Sentient, 2016. 273 p.

174. Dahlke, Rüdiger. *Krankheit als Sprache der Selle: Be-Deutung und Chance der Krankheitsbilder*. C. Bertelsmann Verlag, 2014. 449 p.

175. Dahlke, Rüdiger. *Disease as a Symbol: Psychosomatics - the messages behind your symptoms*. M-Tec, 2000. 552 p.

176. Odoul, Michael. *What Your Aches and Pains Are Telling You: cries of the body, messages from the soul*. Healing Arts Press, 2018. 208 p.

177. Hay, Louise L. *Heal your body: the mental causes for physical illness and the metaphysical way to overcome them*. Hay House, 1995. 83 p.

178. Rainville, Claudia. *La Metamedicina*. Editorial Sirio, 2009. 504 p.

179. Prochaska, James O; DiClemente, Carlos C. The *Transtheoretical Approach: Crossing Traditional Boundaries of Therapy*. Dow Jones-Irwin, 1984. 193 p.

180. Mccullough, Dennis. *My mother, your mother*. HarperCollins, 2009. 263 p.

181. Vieira, Waldo. Técnica da circularidade [verbete]. In: Vieira, Waldo (Org.). *Enciclopédia da Conscienciologia*. 9th ed. Digital. Version 9. Editares, 2018. https://editares.org.br/livro/enciclopedia-da-conscienciologia--9a-edicao/.

182. Vieira, Waldo. Inteligência Evolutiva [verbete]. In: Vieira, Waldo (Org.). *Enciclopédia da Conscienciologia*. 9th ed. Digital. Version 9. Editares, 2018. https://editares.org.br/livro/enciclopedia-da-conscienciologia-9a--edicao/.

183. Kauati, Adriana. "Self-research, parapsychism and self-scientificity. Interparadigmas, ano 2, n. 2, 2014, pp. 21-34. https://www.interparadigmas.org.br/?page_id=88.

184. Vieira, Waldo. Autopesquisologia [verbete]. In: Vieira, Waldo (Org.). *Enciclopédia da Conscienciologia*. 9th ed. Digital. Version 9. Editares, 2018. https://editares.org.br/livro/enciclopedia-da-conscienciologia-9a-edicao/.

185. Cordioli, Cesar. *Calepino Conscienciológico: Coletânea de apontamentos pró-evolutivos*. Editares, 2019. 1222 p.

186. Gaion, Patrícia. "Proposição de metodologia de autopesquisa proexológica". Revista Proexologia, v. 5, n. 5, 2019, pp. 71-80. https://apexinternacional.org/revista/index.php/proexologia/article/view/61/63.

187. Silveira, Fernando Lang da. "A metodologia dos programas de pesquisa: a epistemologia de Imre Lakatos". Caderno Brasileiro de Ensino de Física, v. 13, n. 3, 1996, pp. 219-230. https://doi.org/10.5007/%x.

188. Kauati, Adriana. Autocientificidade [verbete]. In: Vieira, Waldo (Org.). *Enciclopédia da Conscienciologia*. 9th ed. Digital. Version 9. Editares, 2018. https://editares.org.br/livro/enciclopedia-da-conscienciologia-9a--edicao/.

189. Carvalho, Juliana; Carvalho, Francisco. "Síndrome do conflito de paradigmas: proposição de nova patologia consciencial". Conscientia, v. 15, n. 1, 2011, pp. 80-91.

190. Zaslavsky, Alexandre et al. "Self-Paradigmatic transition diagram". Interparadigmas, n. 7, 2020, pp. 109-132. https://www.interparadigmas.org.br/?page_id=746.

191. Balona, Malu. *Síndrome do Estrangeiro*. Editares, 2006. 330 p.

192. Kahneman, Daniel. *Thinking, fast and slow*. Farrar, 2012. 514 p.

193. Sevinc, Gunes; Lazar, Sara W. "How does mindfulness training improve moral cognition: a theoretical and experimental framework for the study of embodied ethics". Current Opinion in Psychology, v. 28, 2019, pp. 268-272. https://doi.org/10.1016/j.copsyc.2019.02.006.

194. Fredrickson, Barbara L. *Love 2.0: Finding Happiness and health moments of connection*. Plume, 2015. 272 p.

195. Marques-Deak, Andrea; Sternberg, Esther. "Psiconeuroimunologia: a relação entre o sistema nervoso central e o sistema imunológico". Revista Brasileira de Psiquiatria, v. 26, n. 3, 2004, pp. 143-144. https://doi.org/10.1590/S1516-44462004000300002.

196. Brown, Brené. *A coragem de ser imperfeito*. Sextante, 2016. 208 p.

197. Brown, Brené. *Mais Forte do que nunca*. Sextante, 2015. 272 p.

198. Brown, Brené. *A Arte da Imperfeição*. Sextante, 2020. 176 p.

199. Vieira, Waldo. Autorrecuperação dos Megacons [verbete]. In: Vieira, Waldo (Org.). *Enciclopédia da Conscienciologia*. 9th ed. Digital. Version 9. Editares, 2018. https://editares.org.br/livro/enciclopedia-da-consciencologia-9a-edicao/.

200. Vieira, Waldo. Autoconsciencialidade [verbete]. In: Vieira, Waldo (Org.). *Enciclopédia da Conscienciologia*. 9th ed. Digital. Version 9. Editares, 2018. https://editares.org.br/livro/enciclopedia-da-conscienciologia-9a-edicao/.

201. Tornieri, Sandra. Taxologia da Autossinalética [verbete]. In: Vieira, Waldo (Org.). *Enciclopédia da Conscienciologia*. 9th ed. Digital. Version 9. Editares, 2018. https://editares.org.br/livro/enciclopedia-da-consciencologia-9a-edicao/.

202. Vieira, Waldo. Reconhecimento [verbete]. In: Vieira, Waldo (Org.). *Enciclopédia da Conscienciologia*. 9th ed. Digital. Version 9. Editares, 2018. https://editares.org.br/livro/enciclopedia-da-consciencologia-9a-edicao/.

203. Vieira, Waldo. Inspiração [verbete]. In: Vieira, Waldo (Org.). *Enciclopédia da Conscienciologia*. 9th ed. Digital. Version 9. Editares, 2018. https://editares.org.br/livro/enciclopedia-da-consciencologia-9a-edicao/.

204. Vieira, Waldo. Marca Parapsíquica [verbete]. In: Vieira, Waldo (Org.). *Enciclopédia da Conscienciologia*. 9th ed. Digital. Version 9. Editares, 2018. https://editares.org.br/livro/enciclopedia-da-consciencologia-9a-edicao/.

205. Vieira, Waldo (Org.). *Enciclopédia da Conscienciologia*. 9th ed. Digital. Version 9. Editares, 2018. https://editares.org.br/livro/enciclopedia-da-consciencologia-9a-edicao/.

206. Wojslaw, Eliane et al. (Orgs). *The english-portuguese glossary of essential Conscientiology terms*. Editares, 2020. 332p.

207. Vieira, Waldo. Trafalismo [verbete]. In: Vieira, Waldo (Org.). *Enciclopédia da Conscienciologia*. 9th ed. Digital. Version 9. Editares, 2018, https://editares.org.br/livro/enciclopedia-da-consciencologia-9a-edicao/.

208. Vieira, Waldo. Autobagagem Holobiográfica [verbete]. In: Vieira, Waldo (Org.). *Enciclopédia da Conscienciologia*. 9th ed. Digital. Version 9. Editares, 2018. https://editares.org.br/livro/enciclopedia-da-consciencologia-9a-edicao/.

209. Vieira, Waldo. Holopensene [verbete]. In: Vieira, Waldo (Org.). *Enciclopédia da Conscienciologia*. 9th ed. Digital. Version 9. Editares, 2018. https://editares.org.br/livro/enciclopedia-da-conscienciologia-9a-edicao/.

210. Vieira, Waldo. Iscagem Interconsciencial [verbete]. In: Vieira, Waldo (Org.). *Enciclopédia da Conscienciologia*. 9th ed. Digital. Version 9. Editares, 2018. https://editares.org.br/livro/enciclopedia-da-conscienciologia-9a-edicao/.

211. Vieira, Waldo. Megaeuforização [verbete]. In: Vieira, Waldo (Org.). *Enciclopédia da Conscienciologia*. 9th ed. Digital. Version 9. Editares, 2018. https://editares.org.br/livro/enciclopedia-da-conscienciologia-9a-edicao/.

212. Vieira, Waldo. Ofiexologia [verbete]. In: Vieira, Waldo (Org.). *Enciclopédia da Conscienciologia*. 9th ed. Digital. Version 9. Editares, 2018. https://editares.org.br/livro/enciclopedia-da-conscienciologia-9a-edicao/.

213. Vieira, Waldo. Parapsiquismo [verbete]. In: Vieira, Waldo (Org.). *Enciclopédia da Conscienciologia*. 9th ed. Digital. Version 9. Editares, 2018. https://editares.org.br/livro/enciclopedia-da-conscienciologia-9a-edicao/.

214. Vieira, Waldo. Princípio da Descrença [verbete]. In: Vieira, Waldo (Org.). *Enciclopédia da Conscienciologia*. 9th ed. Digital. Version 9. Editares, 2018. https://editares.org.br/livro/enciclopedia-da-conscienciologia-9a-edicao/.

215. Vieira, Waldo. Autorretrocognição [verbete]. In: Vieira, Waldo (Org.). *Enciclopédia da Conscienciologia*. 9th ed. Digital. Version 9. Editares, 2018, https://editares.org.br/livro/enciclopedia-da-conscienciologia-9a-edicao/.

216. Vieira, Waldo. Prospecção Seriexológica [verbete]. In: Vieira, Waldo (Org.). *Enciclopédia da Conscienciologia*. 9th ed. Digital. Version 9. Editares, 2018, https://editares.org.br/livro/enciclopedia-da-conscienciologia-9a-edicao/.

217. Vieira, Waldo. Megapensene Trivocabular [verbete]. In: Vieira, Waldo (Org.). *Enciclopédia da Conscienciologia*. 9th ed. Digital. Version 9. Editares, 2018. https://editares.org.br/livro/enciclopedia-da-conscienciologia-9a-edicao/.

218. Vieira, Waldo. Verpon [verbete]. In: Vieira, Waldo (org.). *Enciclopédia da Conscienciologia*. 9th ed. Digital. Version 9. Editares, 2018, https://editares.org.br/livro/enciclopedia-da-conscienciologia-9a-edicao/.

Audiovisual Sources

Live Up to Your Name. Dir. Hong Jong-chan. Perf. Kim Nam-gil and Kim Ah-joong. tvN, 2017.

The Sixth Sense. Dir. M. Night Shymalan. Perf. Bruce Willis and Haley Joel Osment. Buena Bista Pictures Distribution, 1999.

The Others. Dir. Alejandro Amenábar. Perf. Nicole Kidman and Alakina Mann. Dimension Films, 2001.

A Beautiful Mind. Dir. Ron Howard. Perf. Russel Crowe and Jennifer Connelly. Universal Pictures, 2001.

A Pure Formality. Dir. Giuseppe Tornatore. Perf. Gérard Depardieu and Roman Polanski. AFMD; Penta Distribuizone, 1994.

List of acronyms

BME – Basic Mobilization of Energies

CEB – Cultivating Emotional Balance

CI – Conscientiocentric Institutions

CSO – Cosmoethical Sceptical Optimism

DCC – Duo Code of Cosmoethics

EFT – Emotional Freedom Techniques

EI – Evolutionary Intelligence

EMDR – Eye Movement Desensitization and Reprocessing

FEMA – Find-Embrace-Move-Again

GCC – Group Code of Cosmoethics

ICT – Integrative Community Therapy

ICGE – Cognopolitan Institute of Geography and Statistics

Intercongrepics – International Congress of Integrative and Complementary Practices and Public Health

ISIC – Interassistantial Services for the Internationalization of Conscientiology

NDE – Near-Death Experience

NLP – Neurolinguistic Programming

NSAIDs – Non-Steroidal Anti-Inflammatory Drugs

OIC – International Organization of Conscientiotherapy

PCC – Personal Code of Cosmoethics

PD – Principle of Disbelief

PICS – Complementary and Integrative Practices in Health – (Práticas Integrativas e Complementare em Saúde)

PNEI – Psycho-Neuro-Endocrine-Immunology

PNPIC – National Policy of Integrative and Complementary Practices in Health – (Política Nacional de Práticas Integrativas e Complementares em Saúde)

STP – Singular Therapeutic Project

SUS – Unified Health System (Sistema Único de Saúde)

TC – Thought Collective

TCIM – Traditional, Complementary and Integrative Medicines

TS – Thought Style

UFSC – Federal University of Santa Catarina

VHL TCIM – Virtual Health Library on Traditional, Complementary and Integrative Medicines

VS – Vibrational State

WHO – World Health Organization

Glossary

More information about the complementary therapies presented in this book can be accessed at *The Integrative and Complementary Practices in Health Thematic Glossary*[44] and in the official documents of the **World Health Organization**[35-38]. The complementary therapies not described in these documents can be found on the official websites of the associations and institutions that represent them, by searching for the full name of the practices on the internet, especially the National Center for Complementary and Integrative Health website - https://www.nccih.nih.gov/health.

The conscientiological terms used in this book are defined below, based on the definitions in the books *Projectiology*[67], *Encyclopedia of Conscientiology*[205] and *The English-Portuguese Glossary of Essential Conscientiology Terms*[206].

Absentrait: Missing trait in the consciousness' personality. The absent quality in the structure of one's consciential universe that the individual has not yet been able to develop[206:31;219].

Claritask (clari + task): Clarification task. Advanced personal or group assistantial task of elucidation or clarification[67:1099;206:38].

Con: Hypothetical unit of measurement of the level of lucidity of the intraphysical or extraphysical consciousness[67:1099].

Confor (con + for): Interaction between content (idea, essence) and form (appearance, language) in interconsciential communication processes[67:1098; 206:40].

Consciential energy (CE): Energy that the consciousness employs in its general manifestations; the *ene* of thosene[67:1100].

Consciential paradigm: Leading-theory of conscientiology based on the consciousness itself and its attributes[67:1100;206:44].

Consciential self-relay: Advanced condition in which the consciousness evolves by securing one intraphysical existence to another (bound existential programs), like links in a chain, within their multiexistential cycle (holobiography)[67:1100; 206:45].

Conscientiocentric institution (CI): Institution which centers its objectives on the consciousness itself and its evolution[67:1100;206:46].

Conscientiocentrism: Social philosophy which centers its objectives on the consciousness itself and its evolution[67:1100;206:46].

Conscientiogram: Technical form for evaluating the evolutionary level of a consciousness; the consciential megatest whose model is the *Homo sapiens serenissimus*. The basic instrument used in conscientiometric tests[67:1101;206:46].

Conscientiologist: Intraphysical consciousness committed to the permanent study of and objective experimentation within the research fields of conscientiology[67:1101;206:47].

Conscientiology: Science which studies the consciousness in an integral, holosomatic, multidimensional and multiexistential manner[67:1101;206:47].

Conscientiometry: Speciality of conscientiology applied to the study and research of conscientiological measurements, or those related to the consciousness, by using the resources and methods capable of establishing a possible basis for the mathematization of the consciousness. Main instrument: the book Conscientiogram[67:1101;206:48].

Conscientiotherapy: Speciality of conscientiology applied to the study and research of the treatment, relief and remission of consciential pathologies and parapathologies, performed through the resources and techniques derived from conscientiology [67:1101].

Consciex (consci + ex)**:** Extraphysical consciousness; a paracitizen of an extraphysical society. *Outdated variants: spirit, ghost, discarnate*[67:1104;206:49].

Conscin (consci + in)**:** Intraphysical consciousness; the human personality; a citizen of intraphysical society. *Outdated variants: incarnate*[67:1106;206:49].

Consciousness: Individual essence or intelligent principle in constant evolution, also known as individuality, soul, spirit, self and ego, perceived in an integral, holosomatic, multidimensional and multiexistential manner[65;67:1101;206:49].

Consoltask (consol + task)**:** Consolation task. Elementary, primary, personal or group assistantial task of consolation[67:1101;206:50].

Cosmoethics (cosmo + ethics)**:** Ethics or the reflection upon the multidimensional, cosmic moral principles, norms and values, which defines holomaturity, situated beyond all human or intraphysical societal moral principles[67:1101;206:52].

Cosmoethicology: Speciality of conscientiology applied to the study and research of cosmoethics[67:39;206:52].

Desoma (de + soma)**:** Somatic deactivation, near and inevitable for every intraphysical consciousness; final projection; biological death[67:1102;206:56].

Energosoma: Energetic parabody of the human consciousness. *Variant: holochackra*[67:1105].

Evolutionary intelligence: Ability to apprehend, learn or understand and adapt to human life, based on the self-aware theorical application and expansion of the mechanism of the already assimilated consciential, personal evolution[182;206:65].

Existential self-mimicry: Imitation or repetition by an intraphysical consciousness, of life occurrences or past experiences, from present life or previous existences[67:1103; 206:68].

Extraphysical helper: Extraphysical consciousness who aids and assists one or various intraphysical consciousnesses; extraphysical benefactor. *Outdated variants: guardian angel; angel of light; guide; spiritual guide; mentor*[67:1105; 206:71].

Groupkarma (group + karma): Principle of cause and effect acting on the evolution of the consciousness, when centred on the evolutionary group. The state of individual freewill, when linked to the evolutionary group[67:1104;206:76].

Holobiography (holo + biography): Set of the multiexistential and multidimensional experiences of a consciousness across the cycle of personal existences [67:1105;207].

Holomemory (holo + memory): Causal, composed, implacable, multimillennial, multiexistential, uninterrupted, personal memory; which retains all facts relative to the consciousness. *Variants: multimemory, polymemory*[67:1105;206:80].

Holosoma (holo + soma): Set of vehicles of manifestation of the intraphysical consciousness: soma, energosoma, psychosoma and mentalsoma; and of the extraphysical consciousness: psychosoma and mentalsoma[67:1105].

Holosomatic homeostasis: Healthy integrated state of harmony of the holosoma[67:1105;206:81].

Holosomatics (holo + somatics): Speciality of conscientiology applied to the study and research of holosoma[67:1105].

Holothosene (holo + tho + sen + e): Extraphysical atmosphere of aggregated or consolidated thosenes of each consciousness or group of consciousnesses[67:1105;206:83;208].

Interconsciential bait: Condition of an intraphysical consciousness when acting as an energetic bait in order to assist ill extraphysical consciousness[67: 614,695;209].

Intermission: Extraphysical period of the consciousness between two of their physical lives. *Variants: intermissive period*[67:1106;206:88].

Intermissive course: Set of disciplines and theoretical and practical experiences administered to an extraphysical consciousness, after a certain evolutionary level, during the period of consciential intermission, within the cycle of personal existences. The objective of the intermissive course is consciential completism in the next human life[67:1106;206:88].

Intraphysicality: Condition of human, intraphysical life, or the human consciousness' existence[67:1107;206:90].

Lucid projection (LP): Projection of the intraphysical consciousness out of the body. *Variants: conscious projection, out-of-body experience (OBE), extracorporeal experience. Outdated variants: astral projection*[67:1107;206:94].

Macrosoma (macro + soma)**:** Extraordinary or supercustomized soma for the execution of a specific existential program[67:1107;206:96].

Megaeuphorization (mega + euphorization): Energetic state induced by the strong will of a consciousness, by means of a maximum exultation of consciential energies from one's energosphere or holossoma. This leads to the homeostatic apex of the intimate harmonization of one's consciential microuniverse[206:98;210].

Melin (mel + in): Intraphysical melancholy; the condition of intraphysical or *pre-mortem* melancholy[67:1107;206:100].

Mentalsoma (mental + soma)**:** Mental body or discernment parabody of the consciousness[67:1107].

Multidimensional self-awareness (MSA): Condition of mature lucidity of an intraphysical consciousness with respect to life in the evolved state of multidimensionality, attained through lucid projection[67:1108; 206:104].

Offiex: Extraphysical clinic. Extraphysical treatment center of a veteran practitioner of penta[67:1104;212].

Orthothosene (ortho + tho + sen + e)**:** Correct or cosmoethical thosene, pertaining to consciential holomaturity; the unit of measurement of practical cosmoethics, according to conscientiometry[67:1108].

Para: Prefix that means beyond or besides, as in parafact. It also means extraphysical[67:1108].

Paragenetics: Genetics that is inherited by a consciousness from itself. Such genetics relate to all the consciousness' innate traits and temperament, which left their mark from past lives on the consciousness' psychosoma and mentalsoma until the present day[67:1108;206:112].

Parapsychic signal: Existence, identification and self-aware use of personal, animic, parapsychic, energetic signals that every intraphysical consciousness possesses. *Variants: parapsychic sign, parapsychic signage, parapsychic signaletic*[67:1109;206:118].

Parapsychism: Paraperceptions of the consciousness, beyond physical body senses, capable of perceiving energetic, extraphysical or parapsychic phenomena[213].

Pathothosene (patho + tho + sen + e)**:** Pathological thosene or consciential insanity; mental peccadillo; pathological will; sick intention; cerebral rumination[67:1109;206:122].

Penta (p + en + ta)**:** Multidimensional, daily, personal, energetic task that consists of a technical transmission of consciential energies, by an intraphysical consciousness with the continuous assistance of extraphysical helpers directly to other consciousnesses, on a long-term basis or for the rest of one's life. *Outdated variants: passes to the dark, passes-to-the-void*[67:1109;206:123].

Post-desomatic parapsychosis: Psychosis of an extraphysical consciousness that ignores having gone through biological death and still believes to manifest itself in the intraphysical or human dimension[67:320].

Principle of Disbelief: Fundamental and irreplaceable proposition by which conscientiology approaches realities, in general, of the cosmos, in any dimension. It rests on self-experimentation and the refusal of the consciousness to admit any conception in *a priori*, dogmatic way[206:127;215].

Proexis (pro + exis)**:** Existential program. Personal existential program of the intraphysical consciousness, established in the extraphysical dimension before rebirth[67:1103;206:127].

Proexology: Speciality of conscientiology applied to the study and research of the proexis or existential program and its evolutionary effects[67:39;206:127].

Projectiology: From Latin, *projectio,* projection; from Greek, *logos,* treatise. Specialty of conscientiology applied to the study and research of projections of the consciousness and its effects, including the projection of consciential energies[67:1110;206:128].

Recin (rec + in): Intraconsciential recycling or the cerebral renovation of the intraphysical consciousness through the creation of new synapses or interneuronal connections, capable of allowing for an adjustment of the existential program, the acquisition of new ideas, neothosenes and other neophilic conquests by a self-motivated lucid person[67:1106;206:131].

Psychosoma (psycho + soma): From Greek, *psyche,* soul; *soma,* body. The emotional parabody of the consciousness; the objective body of the intraphysical consciousness. *Outdated variants: astral body*[67:1110;206:129].

Retrocognition: From Latin, *retro,* back; *cognoscere,* to know. The perceptive faculty through which the intraphysical consciousness becomes aware of facts, scenes, forms, objects, successes and experiences belonging to the distant past, commonly from a human past life or intermissive period[67:1110;217].

Self-thosene (self + tho + sen + e): The thosene of the consciousness itself[67:1111].

***Serenissimus*:** Consciousness experiencing the full extent of the integral condition of lucid serenism. The evolutionary model for Humanity, technically named *Homo sapiens serenissimus* and popularly named *Serenissimus*[67:43,1105;206:84].

Serenology: Specialty of conscientiology applied to the study and research of the *Homo sapiens serenissimus (Serenissimus)*, their traits, characteristics and evolutionary repercussions[67:43;206:138].

Seriexology: Specialty of conscientiology applied to the study and research of existential seriality, or the cycle of personal existences[67:1111;218].

Soma: Human body; physical body[67:1111].

Strongtrait: Strong point or trait of a consciousness' personality; a positive component of the structure of one's consciential universe that propels the consciousness' evolution[67:1111;206:141].

Symas (sym + as): Sympathetic assimilation of Consciential Energies (CEs), through one's will power, usually with the decoding of the set of thosenes of another consciousness or consciousnesses[67:1111; 206:141].

Symdeas (sym + deas): The sympathetic deassimilation of consciential energies practiced through the impulse of one's willpower, normally through the Vibrational State (VS)[67:1111;206:141].

Theorice (theor + ice): Experience of combined theory and practice, on the part of the intraphysical or extraphysical consciousness[67:1112].

Thosene (tho + sen + e): Practical unit of manifestation of the consciousness, which considers thought or idea (conception), sentiment or emotion, and consciential energy all together and indissociably[67:1112;206:143].

Thosenity: Quality of someone's thosenic consciousness[67:1112;206:144].

Trivocabular megathosene: Maximum synthesis of an idea within a minimal form, in a 3 word mini-sentence[206:144;211].

Vehicle of the consciousness: Instrument or body that enables the consciousness to manifest in intraphysicality (intraphysical consciousness) and in other extraphysical dimensions (projected intraphysical consciousness and extraphysical consciousness)[67:1112;206:146].

Verpon: Leading edge relative truth. A new thosene, new idea, new reality (fact) or parareality (parafact) that definitely exists for a consciousness, according to the Principle of Disbelief, obtained through self-research[206:146;220].

Vibrational state (VS): Technical condition of the maximal dynamization of the energosoma's energies through the impulse of the will[67:1112;206:147].

Weaktrait: Weak point or trait of a consciousness' personality; a negative component of the structure of one's consciential universe that the individual has not yet been able to overcome[67:1112;206:149].

Index

The authors

Born in Florianópolis, Santa Catarina, Brazil, the authors are sisters who cultivate an interest in the multiple approaches to care and health.

Fernanda Cabral Schveitzer was born on September 20th, 1981 and currently resides in Foz do Iguaçu, Brazil. She is a physician, a specialist in occupational medicine from the Brazilian Medical Association/National Association of Occupational Medicine (AMB/ANAMT) and a graduate in Medicine (Federal University of Santa Catarina – UFSC). She has been the manager

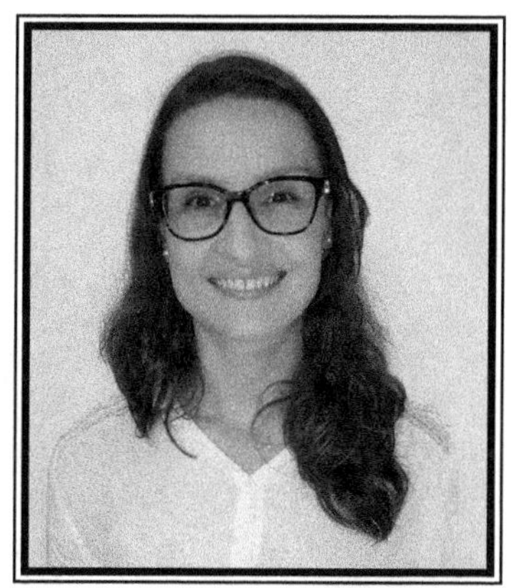

of the Occupational Medicine Division at Itaipu Binacional since 2009, and has been a volunteer of Conscientiology since 1999.

Mariana Cabral Schveitzer was born on July 4th, 1984 and currently resides in the city of São Paulo, Brazil. She is a nurse and university lecturer, with a post-doctorate (School of Nursing at the University of São Paulo – EEUSP). She earned a PhD in Science, double degree (University of São Paulo-Catholic University of Portugal – USP-UCP), and a Master in Nursing (Federal Uni-

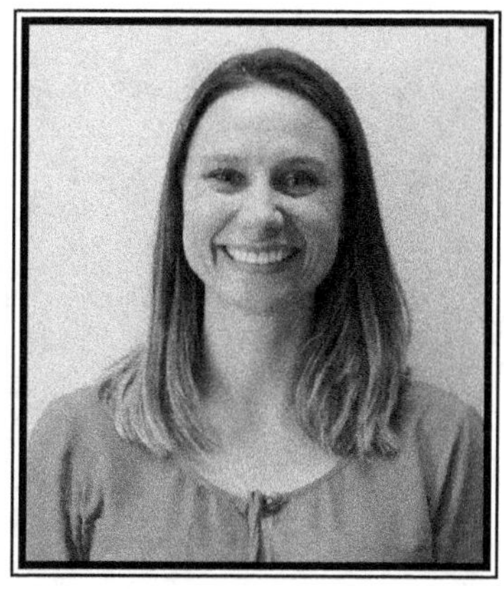

versity of Santa Catarina – UFSC), is specialized in Acupuncture (Faculty of Health Technology – CIEPH-Shandong University), is specialized in Public Health (UFSC) and graduated in Nursing (UFSC). She is currently an Assistant Professor at the Department of Preventive Medicine at the Paulista Medical School at the Federal University of São Paulo (UNIFESP), and has been a volunteer of Conscientiology since 2013.

The translators

Fernanda Lise and Flávia Lise Garcia are mother and daughter, respectively, who were born in Chapecó, Santa Catarina, Brazil. Currently they are living in Pelotas, Rio Grande do Sul, Brazil.

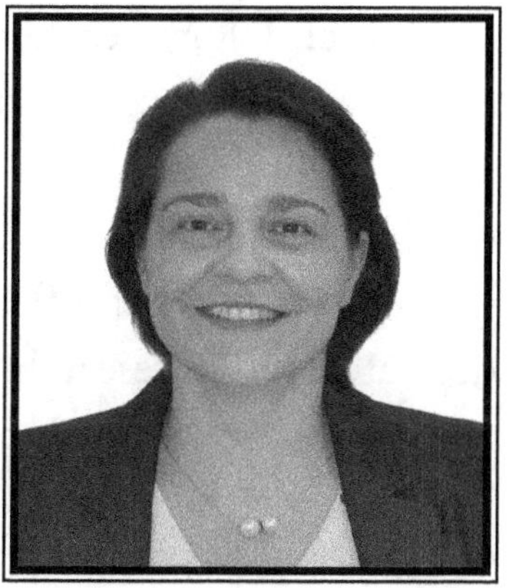

Fernanda Lise is a pediatric nurse (Federal University of Rio Grande do Sul – UFRGS), with a Master and PhD in Science (Federal University of Pelotas – UFPel), a research Scholar at the College of Nursing at Georgia Southern University (GSU), and at the University of Florida (UF). She serves as a member of the International Family Nursing Association (IFNA), since 2017. She is author of the blog www.cuidadoscomfamílias.com.br, which is recognized by the Federal Council of Nursing and the PAHO/WHO as a Nursing Now Brazil initiative. Currently, she is doing post-doc training in Nursing at UFPel.

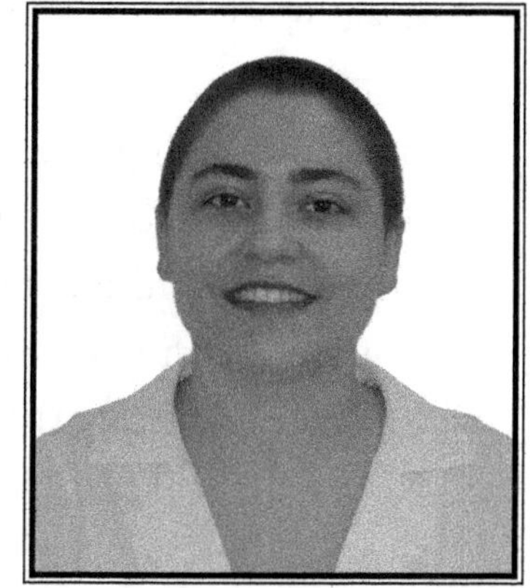

Flávia Lise Garcia studied at Gainesville High School, Gainesville, Florida, US. She is currently undertaking a bachelor's degree in Anthropology at the Universidade Federal de Pelotas (UFPel).

The reviewers

Jaclyn Cowen holds a degree in Urban Planning and a Master's degree in Urban Design. She has been a volunteer of conscientiology since 2007, a conscientiology teacher since 2010 and is currently co-director of ISIC, a non-profit organization with the aim of internationalizing conscientiology, and a volunteer of Consecutivus dedicated to the research of past lives. 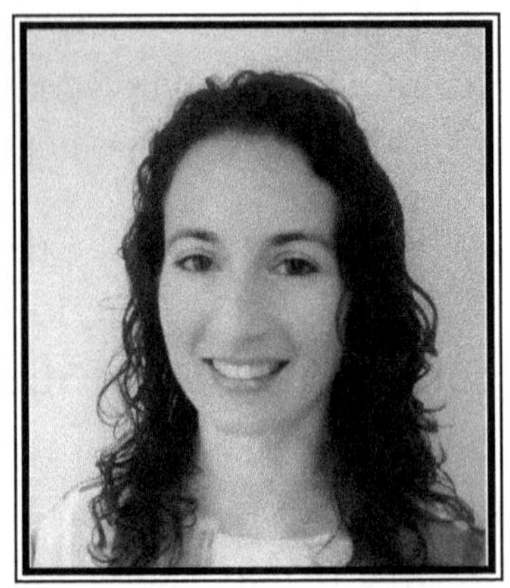 In addition, she is a volunteer of ICNEO, in which she is involved in compiling the English Language Thesaurus of Conscientiology Terminology – ELTHECT. While being based in Sydney Australia most of her life, from 2014, she has been residing in Cognopolis, Foz do Iguaçu.

Victoria Chbane was born in Orlando, Florida, United States of America on July 2nd, 2000. She currently lives in Tampa, Florida, USA. She is presently completing a dual degree in Psychology and Economics, with minors in Statistics and Portuguese at the University of Florida (UF). She is the Vice President of Executive Functioning in the Life Satisfaction and Excellence Lab at the University of Florida, 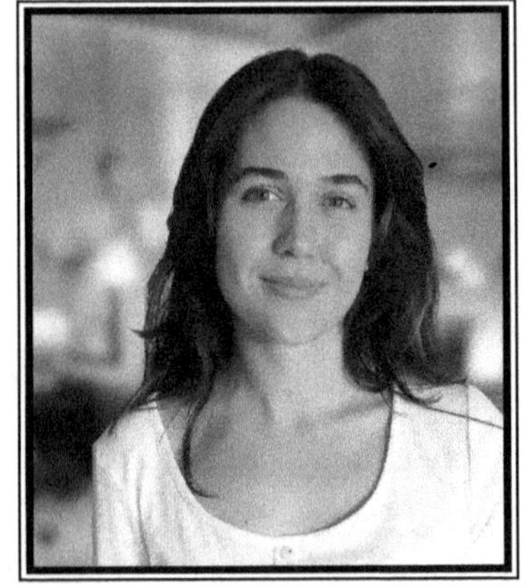

a psychology research lab which studies any topic related to helping individuals achieve life satisfaction and goal achievement. Her future career goals are related to economic research.

Daniel Hiram Zengotita (they/any) is a third-year Political Theory Ph.D. student at the University of Florida in the Department of Political Science. Daniel's research interrogates disparate imaginings of democratic citizenship in the U.S., Brazil, Portugal and the Caribbean. In it, they draw together intertwining-intersecting conversations on affect, judgment, and 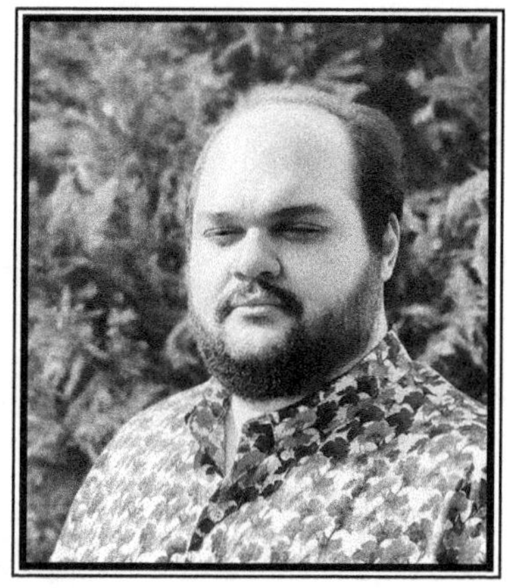 experience to show how historically-marginalized communities contest sexism, homo/transphobia, xenophobia, and racism. Currently, they are researching the relationship between code-switching/language-brokering, language-acquisition, and racialized competency-standards in primary/secondary education and their respective roles in the formation of political judgment. Their research is supported by the Florida Education Fund McKnight Fellowship, the APSA Diversity Fellowship, and the Federal Foreign Language and Area Studies Program at the University of Florida.